THE
ARGININE
SOLUTION

THE
ARGININE
SOLUTION

The First Guide to America's New Cardio-Enhancing Supplement

ROBERT FRIED, Ph.D., and
WOODSON C. MERRELL, M.D.
with James Thornton

WARNER BOOKS

A Time Warner Company

The information herein is not intended to replace the medical advice of your physician. You are advised to consult with your health care professional with regard to matters relating to your health, and in particular regarding matters that may require diagnosis or medical attention.

Copyright © 1999
by Robert Fried, Ph.D., and Woodson C. Merrell, M.D.,
with James Thornton
All rights reserved.
Warner Books, Inc., 1271 Avenue of the Americas,
New York, NY 10020
Visit our Web site at http://warnerbooks.com

 A Time Warner Company

Printed in the United States of America
First Printing: March 1999
10 9 8 7 6 5 4 3 2 1

Library of Congress Cataloging-in-Publication Data

Fried, Robert.
    The arginine solution : the first guide to America's new cardio-
enhancing supplement / Robert Fried and Woodson C. Merrell with
James Thornton.
        p. cm.
    Includes bibliographical references.
    ISBN 0-446-52390-9
    1. Atherosclerotic plaque. 2. Coronary heart disease—
Chemotherapy. 3. Arginine—Therapeutic use. 4. Nitric oxide—
Physiological effect. I. Merrell, Woodson C. II. Thornton,
James, 1952–   . III. Title.
RC692.F75   1999
616.1'23'061—dc21   98-38809
                                                                      CIP

Text design by Stanley S. Drate/Folio Graphics Co., Inc.

*To our colleagues in health care, for being
increasingly open to the potential for safer
and more natural remedies,
and to our patients,
who push us to be more inclined that way.*

Achnowledgments

We would like to thank Alice F. Martell, our agent par excellence and part-time erinaceus zoologist, who championed a book about a little-known biological gas and the amino acid from which our bodies build it. We are very grateful to Alice for her skillful guidance and unwavering belief in this book's potential.

We'd also like to thank Rick Horgan, our editor at Warner Books, for his perseverance and commitment to making *The Arginine Solution* both scientifically rigorous and reader-friendly. From the start, Rick's goal was to make sure the lessons of the laboratory would not be lost on the lay readers whose own cardiovascular health and well-being stood most to benefit.

Our co-writer, James Thornton, a contributing editor at *Men's Journal*, is indebted to his magazine and especially to its health and fitness editor, Mark Jannot, for numerous article assignments on cardiovascular health, sexual function, and related topics, echoes of which both inform and enliven this book.

We also owe a huge debt to Andrei Voustianiouk, our extraordinary research assistant, who helped sort through thousands of research journal articles, extracting the salient details and keeping track of a bewildering inventory of references. We are similarly indebted to Lynn Kasner Morgan, director of the Levy Library, Mount Sinai Medical School, and to Julia Chin, director of the library at Lenox Hill Hospital, a New York University Medical Center affiliate, for opening the doors to Andrei and to us.

Thanks as well to cardiologist Vladimir Shusterman, M.D., a faculty member at the University of Pittsburgh Medical

School, who agreed to review an early version of this manuscript. We also wish to thank the late Charles F. Stroebel, Ph.D., M.D., for his encouragement at the project's outset and for his conclusion, after reading an early draft, that "this book could save hundreds of thousands of lives." It was a quote we kept always close to our hearts, one that helped sustain us throughout the long and not always smooth process of bringing this book to fruition.

We wish to express our gratitude to the following publishers and copyright holders for permission to reproduce charts, graphs, and figures: *Archives of Internal Medicine,* Churchill Livingston/Addison-Wesley Longman, Keats Publishing, and *The New York Times.*

Woodson Merrell would like to thank his wife, Kathy, and his daughters, Caitlin and Isabel, for love, patience, understanding, and encouragement over the last two years of this project.

Bob Fried is indebted to his wife, Virginia Cutchin, for her unwavering cheerfulness during the years that it took to write this book, her faith in the ultimate value of this project, and her diplomatic criticisms of the prose, style, and idiom.

Contents

THE
ARGININE
SOLUTION

1

A Few Grams of Prevention
The New Supplemental Safeguard for Your Good Health

Here's a double health to thee!

—*Lord Byron*

If you're now reading these words, chances are you take your own health, and that of your loved ones, very much to heart. The ancient Greek physician Hippocrates called health "the greatest of human blessings," a sentiment that has been echoed by poets and philosophers throughout the ages. Health is today, as it has always been, the only currency whose presence or absence can make the poor rich, and the rich poor. "Give me health and a day," declared Ralph Waldo Emerson, "and I will make the pomp of emperors ridiculous."

Never before in human history has mankind understood so much about the multiple processes that preserve our well-being, or rob us of it. From genetic engineering to pioneering brain research to potential cures for cancer, we stand poised at the threshold of a new era, a time when countless scourges that have so long afflicted our species are finally beginning to yield to unprecedented scientific investigation. Researchers the world over are increasing the knowledge base at an exponential rate. Sometimes it almost seems as if disease itself has become an endangered species.

1

But the same technological revolution that, with its right hand, forges new hope for cures is, with its left hand, foisting upon all too many of us the need for such cures. Consider this: For our ancestors in antiquity, food was rarely plentiful and obtaining it almost always required great physical effort. Modern life, on the other hand, has put the "ease" into disease. Today, we can lie on the sofa, TV remote control in one hand and cell phone in the other, and dial up a double-cheese pepperoni pizza for speedy home delivery.

The seductiveness of fast food, employment that requires long hours in sedentary pursuits, daily stresses for which the age-old "fight or flight" response can rarely be exercised without inviting trouble, a surfeit of cigarettes and alcohol and various drugs that are all too easily obtainable: These are but a few of the hallmarks of industrialized society for which our hard-scrabble evolution as a species has ill prepared us. No wonder that so-called lifestyle disorders—heart disease, high blood pressure, strokes, diabetes, many forms of cancer, and so on—continue to fell so many of us every year.

Make no mistake: These are hardly overhyped conditions that only target "the other guy." An astonishing 7.5 percent of all American adults alive today have suffered a heart attack or periodic chest pains from heart disease. That's one out of every thirteen adults!

Even as medical researchers look for new ways to undo such damage once it's been wreaked, others look for ways to intercept disease before it's sunk its harpy claws too deeply into our flesh. In recent years, modern medicine has seen a resurgence of interest in integrative medicine—an approach that combines the best of the "fix what's broken" philosophy of conventional modern health care with the "preemptive strike" philosophy long embraced by alternative medicine healers and preventative medicine specialists alike.

Perhaps you, or someone you love, are now suffering from some kind of broken part. Maybe you've been diagnosed with coronary artery disease, high blood pressure, adult-onset diabetes, impotence, or any one of a long list of terribly common health problems. There is nothing like the loss of good health to compel a keen interest in doing everything possible to foster its return.

On the other hand, perhaps you are now in nearly perfect shape, free of any major physiological disorders and totally committed to staying that way. You take seriously the constant drumbeat of caveats and public health advice.

You eat a wholesome diet low in fat and high in fruits, vegetables, and fiber.

You exercise most days of the week, and include both aerobic and strength training in your regimen.

You've quit smoking, or better still, you've managed to avoid ever having suffered an addiction to this most ruinous witches' brew of cynically tailored toxins.

You sleep at least six to eight hours each day.

If you drink alcohol, you do so in moderation.

And to manage the inevitable stresses of life better, you take time for yourself each day to meditate or use other techniques to elicit the relaxation response proven so beneficial in moderating stress hormones.

Perhaps, too, you have also been impressed with the accumulating evidence supporting the health benefits of nutritional therapy—"nutraceutical agents" like vitamins E, C, and the carotenoids; the beneficial omega-3 fatty acids found in coldwater fish; the isoflavones in soy; and a host of other foods, from oat bran to garlic to olive oil, increasingly linked to good health. Other therapeutic agents, especially botanical remedies, are receiving unprecedented scientific study—and being embraced more and more by clinicians and patients alike because of their powerful healing properties.

We will be showing you how a long- and well-known nutrient, the amino acid arginine, is fast emerging as one of the most potent nutraceuticals yet described. It works, when the body breaks it down, in the process releasing a simple gas called nitric oxide, or NO, a substance formerly best known for its presence in smog. In the body, however, NO is hardly a pollutant. Over the last decade, researchers have made a series of truly revolutionary discoveries about the critical functions NO plays in an astonishing array of bodily systems. Indeed, so momentous have these discoveries been, and so far-reaching their implications for bettering human health, that the most prestigious of all scientific awards—the Nobel Prize for Medicine—was bestowed upon three pioneering American NO researchers on October 12, 1998.

Already the work of the three Nobel laureates—Robert F. Furchgott, Louis J. Ignarro, and Ferid Murad—has inspired a legion of pharmacologists searching for new cures for ancient ailments. Case-in-point: the bestselling anti-impotence drug Viagra, which arguably could not have been invented without an understanding of nitric oxide's key role in relaxing the smooth muscles of blood vessels. A wide range of other investigational drugs—designed to treat everything from atherosclerosis to septic shock—may soon hit the market, thanks to the NO discoveries.

Arginine-derived nitric oxide, or ADNO, is a multifaceted molecular marvel, one made all the more amazing by the fact that researchers only so recently discovered that it even exists inside human tissues.

Consider just a sample of the many jobs ADNO has now been shown to perform inside the human body:

- It relaxes arteries, thereby helping to maintain normal blood pressure, which would otherwise skyrocket when ADNO is in short supply.
- It helps keep open the coronary arteries that supply blood to the heart, preventing angina pain.
- It's a potent free-radical scavenger that helps to both lower serum cholesterol and prevent the "bad" LDL cholesterol from oxidizing and becoming even worse.
- It's a powerful anticoagulant, or blood thinner, that helps prevent blood platelets from clumping together into the clots that can cause heart attack and stroke.
- It enhances blood flow to the penis, helping to boost erections.

- It serves as a critical "bullet" by different immune-system cells that use it to kill foreign bacteria and viruses and even shrink or destroy some cancerous tumors.
- It's used by the brain to encode long-term memory and ensure blood flow to brain cells.
- It functions as a "messenger molecule" that allows nerve cells in the body and the brain to communicate with each other.
- It may reduce pregnancy-related hypertension, a potentially life-threatening condition for mother and child.
- It may help regulate insulin secretion by the pancreas, thereby reducing the risk of diabetes.
- It helps control the lung airways, allowing you to breathe easier and avoid common lung disorders.
- It relaxes "hypertonic" sphincter muscles, preventing and healing hemorrhoids and anal fissures.
- It stimulates the body into releasing the all-important human growth hormone (HGH), a key to longevity as well as improvement in body composition by boosting lean muscle mass and bone density while decreasing fat tissue.

Given such powerful and manifold effects, it is perhaps not surprising that ADNO has also been theoretically linked to some medical disorders. We detail these in the book's final chapter and strongly encourage you, if you suffer from one of these maladies, to discuss arginine supplements with your doctor before initiating self-treatment.

For the vast majority of men and women, however, the use of supplemental ADNO as a nutraceutical self-treatment is safe, devoid of side effects, and often startlingly effective in preventing, controlling, and overcoming common causes for ill health.

If you're looking for ways to counter problems already incurred, we invite you to read on to see how the Arginine Solution can play a role in a speedy return toward health. If you are now healthy but ever open to new strategies to preserve the

---

The Arginine Solution: A Simple Prescription

What to take: Inexpensive dietary supplements of L-arginine, available in powder capsules. There are many distributors of arginine products, and it is available in most stores where health products are sold. See the appendix for a list of some of these distributors and their phone numbers.

How much to take: Begin with one gram per day and after several weeks gradually increase to six grams daily if needed.

When to take it: Split each day's dose into three equal parts and take morning, noon, and night. Ingesting the supplement with carbohydrates can prevent minor stomach upset. Try to avoid taking with protein, as this can inhibit absorption.

Word of caution: For most people, the Arginine Solution is safe and devoid of side effects. Check Chapter 14 for certain specific conditions that may contraindicate arginine supplements. And as is the case with any new medical regimen, it's always best to talk things over with your physician first.

---

robust status quo, we invite you, as well, to weigh the considerable evidence in support of ADNO.

An ounce of prevention, so they say, is worth a pound of cure. We wholeheartedly agree with this sentiment, if not exactly with the dosage level prescribed. As you will see in coming pages, when it comes to the Arginine Solution, you don't need nearly an ounce—a modest three to six *grams* of daily prevention is usually plenty for most adults.

Chances are you're already taking in at least this much, if not more, from your diet. Statistics show that most adults obtain over five grams each day from dietary sources including meat, poultry, fish, dairy products, eggs, cereals, nuts, potatoes, and many other foods. Later in this book, you will see how researchers have safely administered thirty to fifty grams or more of arginine intravenously to patients with certain medical conditions—without triggering any major side effects.

Our recommendation, to be sure, is much, much more conservative. Indeed, our "Arginine Solution"—three to six grams taken by mouth in three divided doses per day—represents the average adult's normal intake. At this level, supplemental arginine appears reasonable and is usually safe—and not because the amount is too small to have much of an effect. Quite the contrary: As you will see throughout this book and in the extensive bibliography of scientific literature that follows, a multitude of studies offer compelling evidence that a few grams of prevention can be worth a *ton* of cure.*

Arginine costs relatively little. Given such a modest price and all the benefits it can provide to a variety of your bodily systems, medical economists calculating cost-to-benefit ratios would be hard pressed to find a better health-care bargain available anywhere today.

---

*The manufacturer and distributor of any arginine product are responsible for determining that it is pure and safe to consume when taken as directed. The authors have no control over its production, packaging, and distribution. We can assume no responsibility for the accuracy of claims made by any manufacturer, distributor, or retail merchant regarding purity and safety.

2

Getting to Know NO
The Nitric Oxide Revolution

A simple and familiar chemical best known as a precursor of acid rain and smog is emerging in a surprising new role, as one of the most powerful known substances in controlling numerous bodily functions.

—The New York Times, *July 1991*

Dr. Robert Fried's Story

It was during the summer of 1991 that I first heard about nitric oxide, a gas molecule that the body creates from the amino acid L-arginine. Frankly, the preliminary reports concerning this humble molecule aroused my skepticism as much as my interest. How could such a simple molecule—a single atom of nitrogen bonded to a single atom of oxygen—possibly perform even a fraction of the roles that researchers worldwide were beginning to ascribe to it? Little did I know at the time that in a little less than a decade, three American researchers would win the Nobel Prize for Medicine for their work on elucidating NO's functions.

To be sure, I was hardly alone in my doubts. Even the pioneers in NO research themselves seemed genuinely taken aback by the astonishing breadth of their discoveries. Dr. Michael A. Marletta, for one, told *The New York Times* that the discovery of nitric oxide's multiple biological functions was "a total surprise," adding that when he discussed the subject with fellow scientists, many found it just too unusual to believe. "Some people *still* look at me when they're being polite with a sidelong glance."

Dr. Salvador Moncada, a renowned British medical researcher who was the first to identify the role of NO in relaxing blood vessels, told the *Times*, "People said I was mad. But now, everybody wonders, How could we have missed it?"

At least Dr. Moncada's short-lived case of "madness" put him in good company. William Harvey, the first person to describe blood circulation in the body, was branded similarly "crack-brained" by his fellow seventeenth-century physicians.

Still, the emerging claims for this humble molecule were both eye-opening and eyebrow-raising. Arginine-derived NO, or ADNO for short, seemed capable of:

- Controlling high blood pressure and heart function
- Reducing serum cholesterol and plaque formation
- Promoting the release of the anti-aging human growth hormone (HGH)
- Helping immune-system cells kill infections and stop some cancer cells from dividing
- Improving memory function
- Stimulating erections in men with erectile dysfunction

At this point in my life, my interest in ADNO was largely academic. As a college professor with numerous publications in clinical respiratory psychophysiology, I found myself reviewing the research literature for any other mention of nitric oxide and arginine that I could find.

I anticipated uncovering a few esoteric citations in obscure journals. I did not at all expect what I ended up getting: an ever-burgeoning file that would swell to 10,000 citations over the next few years. And these studies were not to be found in fringe publications—they were most often appearing in some of the world's most reputable medical journals, from *The New*

England Journal of Medicine and *Hypertension* to *Urology* and the American Heart Association's journal, *Circulation*.

The more I read, the more I came to realize that ADNO was not a fluke destined for the trash heap of previously hyped then discarded "miracle drugs." ADNO was the real thing: a potent biochemical mediator with a huge potential for combating chronic lifestyle-related diseases and for enhancing human health.

Two subsequent events catapulted my academic interest in ADNO into the realm of the personal and therapeutic. First, I discovered numerous reports demonstrating that you can increase the amount of beneficial NO available to your body by dietary supplementation of L-arginine. Indeed, weight lifters have been successfully using supplemental arginine for decades to try to boost muscle growth—without any of the harmful side effects of steroid abuse.

Second, my personal physician gave me some sinister, though not altogether unexpected, news. At the age of fifty-five, my blood pressure had climbed well into the danger zone. I also suffered from frequent bouts of tachycardia, in which my heart beat rapidly even at rest.

To bring the cardiovascular symptoms under control, my doctor prescribed a six-month leave from the stress of my professorial duties. He also prescribed beta-blockers, potent drugs that in effect block the action of "fight or flight" hormones in the heart. With this medicine, my heart rate and blood pressure both soon normalized, but it also triggered depression.

With plenty of time on my hands, I went back and reread my ADNO file. In one report, I discovered that supplemental ADNO can lower blood pressure in some patients as effectively as beta-blockers, but without triggering the depression and frequent sexual dysfunction that are all too common side-effects of beta-blocker drugs. I also learned that a safe, conservative dosage of L-arginine is between three to six grams per day—about the same amount most of us are already getting from food.

I began experimenting with this supplemental dosage and

soon found I could wean myself from beta-blockers. If my hypertension spiked back up, I thought to myself, I could always return to the prescription medication. Amazingly, I have never needed to look back.

Indeed, years after taking my last beta-blocker pill, my blood pressure and heart rate have remained completely normal. As I near the age of sixty-three, I'm happy to report that my daily dose of ADNO has kept me feeling great while inducing only one major side effect: an astonishing enhancement of sexual function! (See Chapter 11.)

Bolstered as I have been by the powerful one-two punch of science and confirming personal experience, I began to tell any of my friends and colleagues willing to listen about the tremendous potential I saw in ADNO. It was not always an easy sell. "You're getting 'cured' by a gas in the body?" one faculty colleague asked, elbowing me in the ribs. "You *must* be kidding, right?"

Another health-care professional, when I told him L-arginine was easily obtainable, openly sneered at me. To him, the only medicine worth swallowing is available with a prescription only and costs a fortune. The stuff you get at health-food stores isn't therapeutic; it's mere placebos for "health nuts." I found myself wondering if ADNO might have any beneficial effects on a pathologically closed mind!

Fortunately, I did encounter plenty of thoughtful individuals, from professors to physicians, who read the research and joined me in believing that ADNO can truly benefit human health. Over and over again, I was urged to write a book that would translate the arcane lessons of the research laboratory into a manual that would help almost anyone combat common diseases and stay well.

In 1994, as luck would have it, I found myself discussing ADNO with a friend and colleague, Dr. Woodson C. Merrell, an internist with special interest and expertise in "alternative" or "complementary" medicine. Dr. Merrell is one of this country's foremost authorities of this approach to healing. He teaches it to medical students at Columbia University College of Physicians and Surgeons and is executive director of the Beth Israel Medical Center's new Center for Health and Healing. He is extremely open-minded—and he won't hesitate to use science to validate, or debunk, the efficacy of any new therapy to come down the pike.

As it turned out, Dr. Merrell was keenly aware of the growing body of research regarding ADNO. Just as I had, he'd come to wonder if ADNO represented a great new weapon to help prevent and reverse many of the major acute and chronic diseases suffered by so many Americans. Hypertension, heart disease, strokes, impotence, and many more of the "modern-day plagues" all seemed to have one thing in common: harm caused by the inadequate production of vital nitric oxide gas by different parts of the body.

Our initial conversation was followed by discussions during which we tried to sort out the genuine promise of ADNO from the attendant hype and wishful thinking. We also began to mail each other clippings about ADNO, and later, more detailed research publications. As the evidence became ever stronger, we both came to feel an obligation to get this information out to everyday people whose lives, like my own, stood to benefit so greatly. The result is this book, which we have co-written with health writer James Thornton.

To your continuing good health!

Dr. Woodson Merrell's Story

It's not every day that you encounter a revolutionary change in the basic understanding of human physiology, but that's exactly what confronted me when I first read the work of the pioneers in ADNO research. Dr. Salvador Moncada, for example, first proved that NO was a biologically active molecule. Not too long afterward, Dr. Jonathan S. Stamler and his colleagues at Duke University Medical Center showed that NO binds to hemoglobin, the blood's chemical "magnet" that delivers oxygen to our cells, then ferries carbon dioxide back to the lungs for dis-charging.[1]

What's more, Dr. Stamler and his team convincingly dem-onstrated that NO is not just some passive molecular hitchhiker along for a blood-borne ride. Instead, it serves as the key regula-tor of blood circulation and lung function. Without NO, human life would be impossible.

Unless you're an aficionado of molecular biology, nitric oxide research might seem at best interesting in an esoteric way. But to biochemists and many physicians alike, the discovery of life on Mars could not have been more exciting. This was a landmark change, one that I immediately knew would not only force revisions in standard medical textbooks but would also lead to a sea change in how we as physicians approach many disorders.

As I searched the research journals for further studies on NO, I found more and more evidence that this "simple" gas, which had for so long remained completely unknown in living tissues, played a host of essential roles in the body, from en-hancing circulation to bolstering immunity. I also learned that the amino acid L-arginine, so naturally abundant in proteins and other common foods, is the body's chief source for creating the NO it needs. Up until recently, arginine's only "therapeutic use" had been by bodybuilders trying to boost muscle growth and help the body eliminate ammonia that accumulates as a toxic by-product of muscle building. Might supplemental argi-nine prove to have other advantages as a "nutraceutical"?

A decade ago, most physicians would have dismissed such a question as outright quackery. But the 1990s have seen an ex-plosion of data on the health benefits of everything from vita-min E and coenzyme Q10 to omega-3 in fatty-acid "fish oils" and the polyphenols in green tea. Countless herbal remedies such as Saint-John's-wort, echinacea, and ginkgo, once con-signed to "folk medicine" status, have demonstrated their effec-tiveness and moved virtually into the mainstream. There is simply no longer any question that human health can be affected positively by nutritional therapy, and doctors who ignore this route for promoting wellness do their patients a disservice.

On the other hand, unthinking acceptance of "all things natural" can be an equally serious mistake. As an assistant clinical professor of medicine at Columbia University College of Physicians and Surgeons, I have since 1993 been teaching medical students a course on "integrative" medicine—that is, the pros and cons of *proven* "alternative" treatments like acupuncture and mind-body techniques, not as a replacement for, but as a complement to, conventional Western medicine.

It is an approach I have long embraced in my own role as a private practice internist. Many of the patients I see each day are not sick, but neither are they well. They are instead, like so many of us in the modern industrialized world, "working on getting sick"—i.e., eating poorly, smoking cigarettes, drinking alcohol to excess, and/or leading a sedentary, high-stress lifestyle.

To help my patients improve their health, I believe it's critical to first guide them toward a lifestyle that focuses on disease prevention through a healthy balance of mind, body, and spirit. When illnesses do strike, whenever possible I recommend treatments that empower a patient's own innate healing responses. Prescription medicines, surgery, and other "conventional" medical solutions all have a valid place in this process, but so can meditation, acupuncture, herbal and nutritional therapy, and other well-researched "complementary" therapies.

Indeed, so strongly do I believe in the integrative approach that I've twice given testimony to the U.S. Congress advocating for the consumer's right to access such care. I also serve on the New York State Office of Professional Medical Conduct as an expert in alternative and complementary treatment. When it comes to health, my bottom line is simple: Pragmatism rules. Time and again, my own experience as a clinician and knowledge of research studies have proven to me that many of the so-called alternative modalities are safer, effective, harmonious tools for fostering optimum health.

The more I learned about NO and arginine, the more I

began to wonder if it too might represent a new tool for promoting wellness. Not long after reading about the research of Drs. Moncada and Stamler and many others, I had occasion to refer an asthma patient to my colleague and friend Dr. Robert Fried, who, among other credentials, happens to be one of the nation's leading authorities on biofeedback as a treatment for asthma, migraines, and stress disorders. In the course of our phone conversation, Bob happened to ask me what I thought about the explosion of research into nitric oxide and arginine. I told him that I found it fascinating but that I couldn't yet see any clinical applications.

The next day, Bob sent over copies of several dozen peer-reviewed research studies he'd been collecting since he first heard about arginine-derived nitric oxide, or ADNO as he called it. These studies showed a variety of conditions responding favorably to ADNO treatment. Bob also confided that he personally knew about at least one spectacular "patient success story": his own. He explained that when a standard drug for hypertension had left him depressed, he had opted to try supplemental arginine instead. It was working so well, and with no discernible side effects, that he was convinced many others might benefit as well from such treatment.

In his own clinical practice, Bob has a history of employing innovative measures to treat breathing problems, but only when such measures have been solidly backed up by science. Bob's own Arginine Solution was a perfect example of this—cutting-edge, yes, but safe and surprisingly effective, too.

Four of the most common health problems primary-care physicians see are high blood pressure, high cholesterol, immune dysfunction, and impotence. For each of these conditions, the pharmaceutical industry has discovered powerful medicine capable of significantly improving a patient's symptoms. Unfortunately, most of these powerful drug treatments also carry with them a risk of serious side effects.

Impressed by the studies Bob gave me, not to mention by his own clinical improvement, I began raising the issue of arginine supplementation as a possible treatment for select patients.

Certainly, if a given patient's blood pressure or cholesterol was so high that a stroke or heart attack seemed imminent, I wouldn't recommend arginine instead of conventional medicines. But in patients with mild to moderate problems where the therapeutic window was still open enough to allow for less draconian treatment, I explained what researchers had already discovered about ADNO—and suggested that they might want to include arginine as part of a comprehensive program to see whether it could help reverse the problem without medication.

Given the choice between a pharmaceutical drug and a nutritional supplement, it's not surprising that many of my patients opted for the latter. What was surprising, to me, at least, was how well so many of them did on arginine. Many who suffered borderline to moderate hypertension saw their blood pressure begin to normalize. And for several patients suffering erectile dysfunction, arginine proved to be a potent remedy.

Since these early treatment successes, I have become increasingly impressed that the effects of arginine can be both significant and durable. When I began asking my colleagues who specialize in cardiology, urology, and other fields if their patients were experiencing similar benefits, to my surprise, none of them had ever recommended supplemental arginine, indeed most knew next to nothing about it. They were, to be sure, uniformly well versed in the latest generation drugs, from ACE inhibitors to the so-called statin medicines, thanks to numerous articles in their respective medical journals.

What was so surprising to me was that these selfsame, very conservative, mainstream journals were also running articles on NO and arginine. Alas, for many in the medical field, nutrition continues to occupy a back seat in their awareness. Perhaps it's analogous to a tree falling in a forest when there's nobody around to hear it. Maybe a treatment based on nutrition can never hope to achieve the same fanfare as a drug that's often heavily promoted.

For many patients' sake, I hope this isn't the case. While no remedy—complementary or conventional—is a guaranteed cure-all, the reasoned use of the Arginine Solution is capable of helping many individuals enhance their health in a gentle, safe, and efficacious manner. Maybe now that nitric oxide research has earned the 1998 Nobel Prize in Medicine, it will help to open skeptical eyes and spur wider acceptance. When Bob Fried invited me to join him in writing a book to get this information out to laypeople and physicians alike, I wholeheartedly signed on to the project. We sincerely hope the following pages will contribute to a better understanding of your body's complex functioning—and show you the promise of a great new, natural way to safeguard your health.

3

Your Arginine Ally
An Unsung Hero Proves Its Worth

<hr>

Because they know not the causes of fevers, or of the plague,
or admirable properties of some medicaments, and the
causes why they are so, must therefore these things be
denyed?

—*William Harvey*

We live in an age of exhilarating medical discovery. Scientific breakthroughs occur routinely, and "miracle drugs" rise and fall in popularity like hemline fashion. This book is not about the latest magic bullet that will cure everything that ails you. It is about a natural substance, the amino acid arginine, that has emerged in the past decade as one of medicine's greatest untold success stories—and one of the human body's best allies in its intrinsic quest for wellness.

Since the early 1980s, an explosion of research in laboratories across the globe has revealed a multitude of ways that arginine works with the body's complex biochemistry to help prevent major diseases, and to restore health to those who already suffer from them.

Researchers now know, for instance, that supplemental arginine—available for pennies a day from conventional distributors—can significantly reduce high blood pressure and slash the risk of the blood clots that trigger heart attacks and strokes. It can often lower cholesterol levels almost as well as high-priced statin drugs, and it can keep the so-called bad cholesterol from

18

oxidizing into an even nastier artery-clogging form. Arginine reduces the risk of diabetes and lessens the severity of damage in those who suffer from it.

Arginine appears to trigger the pituitary gland into releasing human growth hormone, the same substance shown to slow, and even reverse, the aging process itself. It can also restore erectile function to impotent men, and very likely enhance sexuality for women as well.

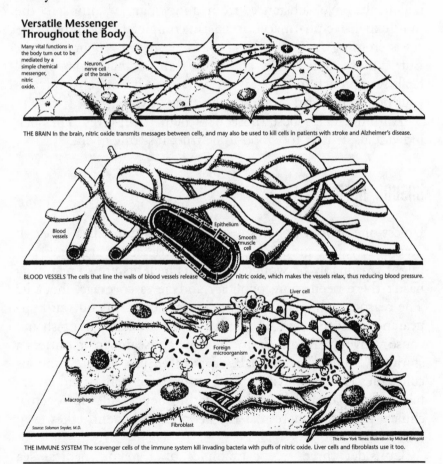

Versatile Messenger Throughout the Body

Many vital functions in the body turn out to be mediated by a simple chemical messenger, nitric oxide.

Neuron, nerve cell of the brain

THE BRAIN In the brain, nitric oxide transmits messages between cells, and may also be used to kill cells in patients with stroke and Alzheimer's disease.

Blood vessels

Epithelium

Smooth muscle cell

BLOOD VESSELS The cells that line the walls of blood vessels release nitric oxide, which makes the vessels relax, thus reducing blood pressure.

Liver cell

Foreign microorganism

Macrophage

Fibroblast

Source: Solomon Snyder, M.D.

The New York Times: Illustration by Michael Reingold

THE IMMUNE SYSTEM The scavenger cells of the immune system kill invading bacteria with puffs of nitric oxide. Liver cells and fibroblasts use it too.

FIGURE 1

Arginine-derived nitric oxide plays a vital role in virtually all body functions. Copyright © 1991 by the New York Times Company. Reprinted with permission.

Other researchers are investigating arginine's role in bolstering immunity, in terms of both fighting off infectious agents and attacking invaders from within, i.e., cancerous tumors. Arginine can boost the brain's ability to store memories and potentially ameliorate a host of other conditions, from acute sickle cell disease to asthma to hemorrhoids.

Sounds too good to be true? It probably is—*if* you believe that taking arginine supplements is all you need to achieve optimal health. No substance, from antioxidant vitamins to the most expensive pharmaceuticals, can completely undo the damage stemming from genetics or a determinedly poor lifestyle. But if those at risk take arginine as an adjunct to an overall healthy approach to living, we're convinced it can help optimize your body's performance in a multitude of ways.

Arginine helps best those who help themselves. For such individuals, it isn't too good to be true; it's truly good.

Unsung Hero

Unless one of your hobbies is keeping up with medical research literature, you've probably heard very little about arginine. You might reasonably be wondering, If its benefits are so real, why hasn't there been more publicity and news coverage about it? The reason is simple: Medical science, despite its outward appearance of cutting-edge topicality, is a remarkably sluggish and conservative organism. From the time a researcher first utters a spirited "Eureka!" in the lab, years often pass before cautious colleagues can be convinced to give up prior beliefs and entertain a new paradigm. And translating new results into actual clinical practice, where real-life people can benefit, takes even longer.

Consider three recent examples of a major medical sea change—and the huge lag time required for initial discoveries to be translated into practical application. Back in the early 1980s, Dr. Barry Marshall, a pathologist at the Royal Perth Hospital in Australia, became convinced that stomach ulcers were not caused by stress but rather by a bacterial infection. He was so sure he'd found the right bug that he made a bacterial milkshake out of *Helicobacter pylori* and drank it. In the long tradition of infectious-disease doctors, Marshall was out to fulfill one of the so-called Koch postulates—i.e., that one way to prove a suspect agent causes a disease is to infect a host with a purified form of it and see if this host gets sick.

Host Marshall got more than he bargained for. Not only did he develop, as he anticipated, a nasty peptic ulcer that lasted for years, but he and fellow researcher Dr. Robin Warren also opened themselves up to nearly two decades of abuse by the medical establishment. Ulcers caused by a bacteria? Absurd! Everyone *knows* that an ulcer, that badge of corporate ascendancy, is caused by stress and too much stomach acid.

But after nearly two decades of die-hard persistence in the face of heckling at scientific conferences, the Australians finally won over their skeptics. Today, there has been a complete revolution in the diagnosis, treatment, and antibiotic cure of many stomach ulcers.

Another famous "heretic" is researcher Dr. Stanley Prusiner, who in the early 1970s became intrigued by a number of devastating brain diseases. One of these was kuru, a horrific condition found in the Fore highlanders of Papua, New Guinea. To honor their dead, tribesmen practiced an odd rite: They ingested the brains of the deceased. Prusiner believed that kuru, along with several other rare human brain disorders such as Creutzfeldt-Jakob disease, had much in common with two neurological diseases affecting animals: scrapie in sheep and mad-cow disease in cattle.

The standard explanation at the time was that all these related conditions were neurodegenerative disorders, that is, the consequence of nerves simply breaking down. But Prusiner had a different idea. His controversial alternative: The nerves were deteriorating because of an infection by tiny particles of protein that lacked DNA or other genetic material. Prusiner called these proteins prions, for "proteinaceous infectious particles." Humans, sheep, and mad cows alike could contract an infection by ingesting prion-contaminated tissues, such as the brains consumed by Fore highlanders.

Other neurologists thought Prusiner was out of his mind. How could such particles, which obviously weren't alive, function like live organisms? So outlandish was Prusiner's proposal that he often couldn't even find a forum to present his work; nobody would listen to him. Indeed, recalls one neurologist, it took Prusiner nearly twenty years of being treated as a pariah by the medical establishment before his idea finally gained acceptance. Prusiner was awarded the Nobel Prize for Medicine in October 1997—one of the few instances in modern times when a researcher working alone, as opposed to a team, has won this award.

One more famous example of a vindicated pariah was Dr. Kilmer S. McCully, who in the late 1960s was widely considered a rising star in medical research. In 1969, he implicated a blood-borne protein metabolite called homocysteine as a major contributing factor in the development of atherosclerosis, or hardening of the arteries. His publications along these lines, however, earned him only widespread criticism and scorn by colleagues. He was forced to toil in virtual anonymity for nearly three decades. Only recently has McCully's theory been vindicated and his reputation resurrected.[1]

In the Gap

In many regards, arginine and nitric oxide research found itself in a similar position—hanging in the gap between initial discovery and widespread acceptance. Over the past decade, the true heroes in the field, pioneers like Drs. Robert F. Furchgott, Louis J. Ignarro, Ferid Murad, Solomon H. Snyder, Salvador Moncada, M. W. Radomski, Jonathan S. Stamler, and R. M. J. Palmer, could hardly have been described as household names. But thanks to the insights they made and continue to make, each of these scientists had become increasingly celebrated in medical circles.

Indeed, Drs. Furchgott and Murad received the highly prestigious 1996 Lasker Award in Basic Medical Research. The journal *Science* made the announcement in October of that year:

The Albert and Mary Lasker Foundation presented this year's awards on 4 October to pioneers in the discovery of nitric oxide's role in the body. Two scientists who helped discover that the toxic chemical nitric oxide also serves as a messenger between cells share the basic medical research awards: Robert Furchgott, distinguished professor emeritus at the State University of New York Health Science Center at Brooklyn, and Ferid Murad, former president and CEO of Molecular Geriatrics Corporation in Lake Bluffs, Illinois.[2]

The editors of *Science* went on to add that the Lasker Award is the most distinguished recognition for biomedical research short of the Nobel Prize for Medicine. At the time, many observers believed that this honor, as well, was only a matter of time. In 1997, Dr. Moncada, working out of London, and Dr. Snyder, at Johns Hopkins University in Baltimore, were both cited by the Institute for Scientific Information as being among the dozen most influential scientists in the world, serious contenders for the Nobel Prize. Think of it—two of the world's top scientists, and both of them involved in NO research. Many in the world of medical and physiological research began to wonder not if but when and who would receive the field's top prize.

On October 12, 1998, the suspense ended: Drs. Furchgott, Ignarro, and Murad were jointly named by the Karolinska Institute as winners of the Nobel Prize for Medicine. These men, of course, represent only the tip of the arginine-research iceberg. Since 1990, nearly 10,000 articles relating to the physiological benefits of arginine have been published in peer-reviewed medical journals. "Peer review" means that studies must be scrupulously designed and stand up to expert scrutiny before being accepted for publication. The journals in question include some of the most famous—and most trusted—in the world, including:

- *The American Journal of Hypertension*
- *The American Journal of Physiology*
- *Annals of Internal Medicine*
- *Cardiology*
- *Circulation*
- *Hypertension*
- *The Journal of the American Medical Association*
- *The Journal of Clinical Investigation*
- *The Journal of Immunology*
- *The Lancet*
- *Nature*
- *The New England Journal of Medicine*
- *Proceedings of the National Academy of Sciences (USA)*
- *Science*
- *Urology*
- And many dozens more

As clinical health-care professionals who, respectively, specialize in treating breathing disorders and internal medicine, our own academic interest was provoked when the early work on arginine first started surfacing. But as more and more of these rigorously designed studies accumulated, our initial interest gave way to increasing excitement. We became ever more convinced that arginine is not a fad or a flash-in-the-pan nutrient destined soon to join yesteryear's failed hyped hopes. Rather, we began to see its very real potential for benefiting the lives of our patients *and* ourselves.

Inexpensive Efficacy

To be sure, we're not the only ones fascinated by the therapeutic possibilities of arginine. Major drug companies in the United States and abroad have launched scientific efforts to develop drugs to boost or inhibit the production of an enzyme the body uses to unleash the power of arginine. Pharmaceutical giants such as Glaxo-Wellcome, Ciba-Geigy, Cassella, Hoechst, and

Merck are all working on ways to use arginine derivatives to combat heart disease, stroke, cancer, asthma, rheumatoid arthritis, impotence, AIDS, and many more conditions.

Kiplinger's Personal Finance Magazine recently reported that the Texas Biotech and Genetech corporations are jointly developing a new arginine product that dissolves blood clots. Yet another company, Comedicus, Inc., is testing TriNORx, an arginine-derived compound intended to prevent arteries from reclogging. Still others are working on arginine salves and ointments that, when rubbed on cold hands and feet, are said to bring warmth by stimulating extra blood flow to the extremities.

Such products notwithstanding, the fact is that arginine is a natural compound and not a new invention—and therefore it has both a downside and an upside. Arguably, drug companies may be less motivated to invest heavily in arginine-derived medicines because of the likely inability to obtain patent protection. On the other hand, arginine is readily available and cost effective—well within the budget of anybody concerned about health. You definitely don't have to mortgage your house to afford it.

Not that you should make the mistake of thinking that "cheap" compounds work less well than the high-priced "new and improved" formulations so heavily advertised in trade and consumer publications. Case in point: One of the few unanimously agreed-upon "miracle drugs" known to mankind costs only a few pennies per tablet. Its name? Aspirin. Ever since the ancient Romans first discovered pain and fever relief by chewing on willow bark, people have been relying on aspirin's active ingredient, salicylic acid, for a host of ailments (including the prevention of colon cancer and second heart attacks). And despite feverish efforts by major drug companies, few of the new "nonsteroidal antiinflammatory" drugs have been proven to work better than aspirin to relieve pain and inflammation.

If you suffer from hypertension, odds are that you probably know about another high-profile example where cheaper is at least as good as, and often better than, "the latest and greatest" drug advances. In its recent report, the Joint National Committee for the Detection, Evaluation, and Treatment of High Blood Pressure strongly recommended that patients requiring medication start with older mainstay treatments like diuretics (water pills) and beta-blockers.[3] Though newer drugs such as calcium channel blockers can play a role in the treatment of select patients, their much greater cost, potential side effects, and the lack of demonstrated superiority all add up to one conclusion: Paying more does not necessarily mean getting more. Indeed, the least expensive approach of all requires no drugs of any sort and often proves maximally effective in treating blood pressure and heart disease: the combination of vegetarian diet, exercise, and meditation long advocated by Dr. Dean Ornish.[4]

As you will read later in this book, patients with high blood pressure now have an even more benign, alternative "drug" therapy that is both effective and inexpensive: arginine.

Risk-Benefit Ratio

Perhaps the oldest tenet of biomedical ethics is this: Above all else, do no harm. Physicians and patients alike must constantly weigh the benefits of any treatment against its risks. When healers swear by the Hippocratic oath, they promise that:

> I will follow that system of regimen which, according to my ability and judgment, I consider for the benefit of my patients, and abstain from whatever is deleterious and mischievous. I will give no deadly medicine to anyone if asked, nor suggest any such counsel.

Unlike synthetic medications formulated by pharmaceutical scientists—drugs that sometimes kill germs and cancer cells by almost killing the patient, too—arginine is a wholly natural substance that you undoubtedly already "take" in your daily diet. With only a few possible exceptions, arginine's side-effect profile is almost completely benign. Adding a few extra grams to what you're already receiving is neither "deleterious" nor "mischievous."

But if the risks are negligible, what about the benefits? To date, results emerging from medical laboratories worldwide—results gleaned from a wide array of animal and human studies—are extremely encouraging. We're convinced that in coming years the 1990s will be remembered by medical historians as the time medicine made a major breakthrough: the discovery of the Arginine Solution.

To be sure, you don't have to wait for the conservative medical establishment's overly cautious acceptance of new ideas to begin benefiting from arginine. If you already suffer from one of the disorders that arginine can relieve, or if you simply want to preserve your health by avoiding such diseases in the future, you owe it to yourself to learn more about arginine today. Even if it proves only fractionally as effective as researchers now believe it to be, arginine represents a major advance in complementary care. Think of it, if you like, as an inexpensive health-insurance policy.

Arginine derives from the Greek word *arginoeis,* meaning "bright." As you'll see in coming chapters, whoever named it "bright" was right on target.

4

Let the Circle Be Unbroken
How Arginine Promotes Your Blood Circulation

When the disease is stronger than one's natural resistance, medicine is of no use. When one's resistance is stronger than the disease, the physician is of no use. When the two factors are balanced, the physician is called in to increase one's natural powers of resistance and assist him to oust the disease.

—*Aphorism of Al-Razi, quoted by Moses Maimonides*

It's hard to be alive in the twilight of twentieth-century America and not worry about your health. We're bombarded daily with dire statistics and newly discovered risk factors. If flesh-eating strep doesn't get you, there's always the hantavirus, car jacking, El Niño–spawned flash floods, drug-resistant tuberculosis, or any other affliction in a seemingly inexhaustible parade of novel, media-darling agents of death.

Now for some good news: You really don't need to worry about the vast majority of these things. Cross them off your worry list; banish them forever from your mind! The odds of actually succumbing to any of these exotic reapers are infinitesimal. Sure, it *can* happen. You *can* also win the $40 million lottery jackpot. But take our word for it, you probably won't.

Now for some less reassuring news: There is one thing you should be taking very seriously—the health of your cardiovascular system, that dynamic marvel of heart, lungs, arteries, veins, and capillaries that circulates blood constantly through every corner of your being. We're not talking about some vague, theo-

28

retical threat now. Heart and blood-vessel disease will eventually kill nearly half of all of us.

Our circulatory system has evolved into a vast network of red streams and tributaries that continually deliver oxygen and nutrients to all our cells, then ferry away wastes and by-products for disposal.

Operating properly, our circulatory system can easily give us ninety or more years of trouble-free, high-quality living. From cradle to grave, a healthy heart, roughly the size of your fist, will pump an average of 75 beats per minute, 4,500 beats per hour, 108,000 beats per day, 39 million beats a year—for a grand total of over *three billion* beats in a lifetime. Depending on what kind of physical shape you're in and what activity you're engaged in, each of these beats can propel anywhere from a few ounces of blood to nearly a soda can's worth on its circular route around your body.

Your arterial blood vessels, in turn, are not mere passive pipes through which blood courses, but rather, active, living organs that work in precisely coordinated ways to keep the circulatory momentum going. As you'll soon learn, even the red blood cells themselves are active participants in the process, emitting a chemical signal that directs the vessels to open or constrict as needed.[1] When every aspect of the system is healthy, each component, from the heart to hemoglobin to the smooth muscles wrapping the most slender of arterioles, will do its miraculous job indefatigably and without complaint.

But as rugged and resilient as the circulatory system is, it is definitely not invulnerable. Many people have genetic factors that produce premature stiffening of the blood vessels. Years of cigarette smoking, a high-fat diet, sedentary living—these are just a few of the chronic lifestyle factors that can degrade, pollute, occlude, and generally break down the circle of life within us all. Undoubtedly, you know by rote the important steps that public-health experts preach to safeguard this circle within: Don't smoke, eat right, get plenty of exercise, reduce stress. As you will see in coming pages, scientists have recently discovered a new, natural way to further help your heart and vasculature remain in top condition.

As our book cover plainly declares, the Arginine Solution can:

- Open clogged arteries
- Lower blood pressure and cholesterol
- Reduce your risk of heart disease and stroke
- Improve your immune system and more

We will soon be describing a few of the fascinating mechanisms through which arginine is able to work such wonders. But first take a few more moments to consider what's truly at stake when you allow your circulatory system to become damaged.

At the risk of sounding a bit morbid, imagine for a moment that you live in a city with a population of exactly 2,278,994 citizens. According to the National Center for Health Statistics, this is precisely the number of Americans who died from all causes in 1994, the most recent year for which such mortality data is currently available. What manner of Grim Reaper do you think got to all these folks?

The overwhelming choice for Public Enemy Number One was heart disease, responsible for killing 361,276 men and 371,133 women. Who says only men need to fear heart disease? It actually kills more women than men.

Cancer felled another 280,465 men and 253,845 women—though increasing rates of cigarette smoking among younger women promise soon to close and maybe even reverse the cancer gender-gap.

The third leading cause of death brings us back again to the circulatory system—not clogged hearts this time but clogged brains. Cerebrovascular disease, aka strokes, killed 60,225 men and 93,081 women. Now factor in deaths by diabetes and atherosclerosis, two other diseases that wreak havoc on blood vessels, and you find that an astonishing 42 percent of all deaths in the United States are directly attributable to disorders of circulation.

All remaining killers, from car wrecks to homicide to HIV, pale in comparison to circulatory disorders. The next time you find yourself watching the evening news and worrying about the crime rate or Ebola virus, realize that the real villain to worry about may be a lot closer than you think—not the bad guys on TV, but the trans fats oiling the potato chips in your hand.

Adding Years to Life—And Life to Years

Heart and vessel diseases don't just imperil your life, they can also take a tremendous toll on the quality of your life. Strokes and heart attacks, for example, are among the leading causes of long-term, chronic disability. Even if you manage to avoid such dire events, a circulatory system clogged with cholesterol, afflicted with hypertension, or constantly keyed up by stress can turn even the simplest activities into an ordeal. What kind of life is it when walking up a short flight of stairs leaves you huffing for breath, or when wrestling with a five-year-old triggers exhaustion?

Inadequate blood supply is now known to be the major cause of another problem that makes quality of life difficult: impotence. Up to 90 percent of all cases of impotence, once thought to be predominantly a psychological problem, are now known to be directly related to "vascular insufficiency"—i.e., the inability to pump enough blood where you need it to go to pump you up.

But men aren't the only ones whose sex lives can be hampered when the hydraulics of passion loses its oomph. Studies conducted in sleep laboratories have long shown that during dream sleep, healthy women also go through repetitive cycles of vaginal blood engorgement parallel to the blood-flow pattern that triggers nocturnal erections in healthy men. Though more research clearly needs to be done, it appears likely that "vascular insufficiency" in women may also hamper satisfying sexuality.

It *is* true that the incidence of deaths from heart disease escalates sharply with advancing age, but it would be a mistake to assume that you're safe just because you're still under age sixty-five. Consider: Autopsies of young soldiers who died in combat during the Korean Conflict revealed that many already suffered fatty streaks in their heart arteries. To be sure, a fatty streak at age twenty can blossom in just a few short decades into a ragged, calcified plaque that's a springboard for blood clots. But even if you luck out and avoid such a fate, less than clean pipes can translate into a less than vigorous, robust life.

Perhaps you've already joined the millions of men and women who have been diagnosed with one of the cardiovascular scourges so rife in our couch-potato culture: clogged arteries, high blood pressure, skyrocketing cholesterol, even aptly named CAD (coronary artery disease) itself. Perhaps heart disease runs in your family, and you feel as though your heart's beats sound like the ticking of a time bomb. Or maybe you're in great shape, a devoted exerciser who's so far managed to steer clear of any circulatory system problems—but you're wondering just how long your luck will hold.

Though there is some "luck" involved in cardiovascular health, vis-à-vis the genetic roll of the dice, genes are only an influence, not a determinant. There's no rational reason for fatalism. Some people with a strong family history of cardiovascular disease may see progressive hardening of the arteries as their inexorable fate—as certain as death and taxes. But this is just not true. Thanks to the pioneering work of researchers such as Dean Ornish, M.D., atherosclerosis has clearly been shown to be not only preventable but even reversible with diet, exercise, smoking cessation, and stress management.[2] There's no question that making such wise choices today is the smartest thing you can do to ensure your long-term cardiovascular health.

But if you're already doing all the right things and you want to do more, there's a revolutionary new way to help optimize the performance of your circulatory system. It's called arginine, a natural food substance that provides the cardiovascular system with the raw material needed to make a key chemical signaler.

Ever-mounting evidence strongly suggests that those who

avail themselves of the Arginine Solution can rejuvenate their circulatory systems, reversing damage already done and setting the stage for continued good health well into the future.

ADNO

Arginine is an amino acid, that is, one of twenty-two "building blocks" that make up the proteins that are required by nearly every living cell. In fact, half the dry weight of our cells is made up of proteins, which makes protein the single most common class of biological molecule on earth. Your muscle cells, the enzymes that catalyze biochemical reactions, the collagen that makes up your skin and connective tissue, the insulin that regulates blood sugar, and even the hemoglobin that carries oxygen in your blood are just a few examples of proteins in action. Arginine participates in all of these critical activities, plus it detoxifies your body by helping your liver eliminate ammonia, a deleterious waste product that can build up rapidly during heavy lifting, sprinting, and other short but explosive bouts of exercise.

Arginine performs another critical function not shared by any of its amino-acid cousins. It can be broken down to produce nitric oxide, or NO, a gas that lasts no more than a few seconds at a time but which scientists now know is one of the single most critical molecules in the body. (Just for the record, NO is *not* nitrous oxide, aka the laughing gas your dentist may use as an anesthetic. It *is* one of the components of Los Angeles smog, which goes to show you that something so good in moderation can have less salubrious effects in excess.)

Arginine comes in two mirror-image forms, identical except for their molecular orientation, much like your left and right hand. So-called L-arginine, the left-handed molecule, is the body's primary source for NO. For shorthand purposes throughout the rest of this book, we will be referring to it as ADNO, that is, L-arginine-derived nitric oxide. NO can also be synthesized from other nitrogen-containing compounds, such as nitrates and nitrites, but usually it comes from the amino acid L-arginine, the same compound found in many foods as well as in capsule supplements available at pharmacies and stores where health foods are sold.

We may occasionally sound like ADNO evangelists, but the truth is, we can hardly help ourselves. We are constrained by the limitations of a book such as this to confine ourselves to the more important aspects of what nitric oxide does in the body.

The more than 10,000 research articles that have appeared in medical journals and textbooks since the biological role of nitric oxide was discovered in the 1980s clearly show that *"absolutely everything in the body depends on it."* No one could have put it better than Dr. Jonathan S. Stamler, professor of medicine at Duke University Medical Center, Durham, North Carolina, when he was quoted in 1996 in *The New York Times* as saying:

> It does everything, everywhere. You cannot name a major cellular response or physiological effect in which [ADNO] is not implicated today. It's involved in complex behavioral changes in the brain, airway relaxation, beating of the heart, dilation of blood vessels, regulation of intestinal movement, function of blood cells, the immune system, even how digits and arms move.[3]

In the chapters that follow, you'll learn much more about the properties and benefits of ADNO for treating specific disorders. You'll also see how the Arginine Solution can help keep your system fine-tuned and running smoothly, in the process helping to preserve current health and preempt future problems.

If you have already been diagnosed with a specific medical disorder that ADNO can treat, feel free to skip ahead to learn more about new hope for what ails you. Otherwise, take a moment to read about the history of ADNO research—a fascinating medical mystery story that promises a happy ending for anyone concerned about health.

5

From Nitro to ADNO
A Medical Mystery Solved

It helps maintain blood pressure by dilating blood vessels, helps kill foreign invaders in the immune response, is a major mediator of penile erections, and is probably a major biochemical component of long-term memory . . . [these are] just a few of its benefits.

—*The editors of the highly prestigious journal* Science, *after voting nitric oxide the 1992 Science Molecule of the Year*

Nearly a century before researchers discovered ADNO, clues about its existence were already beginning to emerge. You may have heard that patients with coronary artery disease often suffer angina pectoris, a severe, radiating form of chest pain that's caused by a spasm of the coronary vessels that straddle the heart. You may also know that nitroglycerin—the same active ingredient found in dynamite—can bring prompt relief to angina sufferers.

In the past, nitroglycerin was given as a pill placed under the tongue, where it rapidly dissolved and entered the bloodstream. Today, many patients wear nitroglycerin skin patches on the chest, near their heart. Regardless of the route of administration, doctors now know that nitroglycerin works by rapidly dilating blood vessels, allowing more blood and oxygen to reach the starved heart muscle. The exact biochemical mechanism behind this dilation, however, remained elusive until only recently.

Ironically, dynamite was invented by a Swedish pacifist whose goal was to make explosives safer to handle, a feat he

35

accomplished by mixing the highly unstable nitroglycerin with an absorbent substance. The inventor's name was Alfred Bernhard Nobel, and he felt so ambivalent about his profitable brainchild that in his will he endowed annual prizes in the sciences, literature, and the promotion of international peace. What began in the nineteenth century with a nitrogen-related bang was destined to come full circle with a nitric oxide–related Nobel Prize in Medicine.

Another clue on the path to ADNO was uncovered in 1918. Again, it involved a substance that, like nitroglycerin, is deadly in excess but therapeutic in low doses. The drug in question: cyanide, a potent poison that smells like bitter almonds and kills by depressing respiration. In much smaller doses, however, this nitrogen-containing compound has the opposite effect—it actually stimulates respiration. The problem was that giving patients enough cyanide to benefit them but not so much as to kill them required walking a tightrope. For this reason, cyanide was largely dismissed as a medicine by the late 1800s, except for trace amounts in some cough medicines.

But four Wisconsin physicians who were treating severely ill psychiatric patients decided that cyanide had had undeserved bad press. After establishing safe levels for its injection, they tested it on ten people diagnosed with schizophrenia who were also suffering from advanced heart and lung disease. For short periods of time following treatment, the patients improved both physically and mentally.

The authors of this study, who published their findings in the *Archives of Internal Medicine,* noted that one patient who had endured frequent seizures became seizure free for the first time following cyanide injection. In another patient, the transformation was even more astonishing.

As the authors wrote:

> The most interesting instance of psychic stimulation was observed in case 10. This patient, who had dementia praecox [schizophrenia], entered the hospital June 27, 1917, and up to the time of the injection had not spoken a word, so that no

history was obtainable except from the meager statement on his commitment papers. After receiving an injection of 102 c.c. of fiftieth-normal sodium cyanide within a period of sixty-four minutes, the patient conversed, answered questions and attempted to explain his prolonged silence.[1]

It would take almost seventy more years before researchers would learn the complex roles that nitric oxide plays in everything from circulation to immunity to nerve and brain function. We now know that cyanide is a nitric oxide donor. Arguably, the Wisconsin experiment is the first published incidence of NO therapy—though nearly three-quarters of a century would elapse before this bizarre experiment would make any theoretical sense.

The Discovery of EDRF

Despite tantalizing clues that substances the body uses to make nitric oxide—NO donors like arginine, nitrates, nitroglycerin, and even trace amounts of cyanide—were doing *something* beneficial to human physiology, the medical mystery would remain unsolved until nearly the end of the twentieth century. Indeed, it wasn't until the 1980s that researchers even began to suspect that there even *was* a mystery. Once solved, years more would pass before conventional medicine finally acknowledged the validity of the solution.

One key line of evidence emerged from researchers studying two of the body's most important hormones. One of these, commonly referred to as adrenaline (epinephrine), is the body's "upper"—it triggers your heart to beat faster, your blood vessels to constrict, your bowels and bladder to jettison their cargoes, and a variety of other physiological changes all orchestrated to help you better fight or flee a threat. Without adrenaline, we would all arguably be a lot calmer—assuming we survived the perils of the world at large.

A sort of reverse adrenaline is called acetylcholine, an inhibitor of the same "fight or flight" responses that adrenaline triggers. Without acetylcholine, we would be forever keyed up and on edge. *Semper paratus* may be a fine motto for the Boy Scouts, but when it comes to the human body, being always prepared, even when there is no threat on the horizon, can be as damaging to health as being forever unprepared. Adrenaline and acetylcholine, therefore, work hand in hand, juicing us up when necessary, then letting us relax when a threat has passed.

For many years, scientists studying acetylcholine had been perplexed by a seeming paradox. When administered to living subjects, acetylcholine usually produced a potent blood-vessel relaxing effect, precisely as expected. But when administered to strips of dissected tissue, it occasionally had the opposite effect, i.e., the "relaxing" hormone would trigger the same vascular constriction caused by adrenaline.

In 1980, Dr. Robert F. Furchgott and his colleague Dr. John V. Zawadzki performed an experiment at the Downstate Medical School in Brooklyn, New York, in which they witnessed this paradox firsthand.[2] After applying acetylcholine to strips of rabbit blood vessel cultured in a Petri dish, they expected to observe dilation but instead found constriction. How could this be?

What Drs. Furchgott and Zawadzki eventually discovered was the key role played by a layer of specialized cells called endothelial cells that line the innermost surface of blood vessels. Previous researchers had assumed that the endothelium played at most a minor and passive role in relaxing blood vessels. And so, during the "preparation" of tissue samples for study, the endothelium was often unintentionally rubbed away.

Drs. Furchgott and Zawadzki were the first to challenge the assumption that the endothelium plays no special role in blood vessel control. A series of experiments eventually led them to an important new insight: The *endothelium must be intact* if the blood vessels are to respond to acetylcholine with relaxation. The implications of this conclusion were startling and revolutionary: Acetylcholine, they realized, does not directly dilate arteries but instead signals a mysterious and unidentified substance made by endothelial cells that actually triggers the dilating. Damaging the endothelium prevents production of this unidentified relaxing substance, which the research team quickly dubbed EDRF, for "endothelium-dependent relaxing factor." This discovery set conventional thinking in cardiovascular physiology on its head and triggered a worldwide search for the molecular identity of the mysterious EDRF.

NO Wonder: From EDRF to Molecule of the Year

This identification was finally and conclusively made by British medical researchers—principally, Drs. Salvador Moncada, R. M. J. Palmer, and E. Annie Higgs—who proved that endothelium-dependent relaxing factor (EDRF) was in fact nitric oxide, a short-lived gas that endothelial cells synthesize primarily from arginine but also from nitrates and nitrites.[3]

Follow-up experiments also showed that when blood-vessel strips are deprived of oxygen, they constrict as expected, but when these same oxygen-deprived strips are provided with nitrates, they relax. The reason: Nitrates provide more of the raw materials that the endothelial cells need to make NO. No wonder nitroglycerin and cyanide both had beneficial effects—they boost production of the nitric oxide needed to relax blood vessels.

Despite this and other lines of evidence, not everyone in the research world immediately accepted the idea that such a simple molecule, one that lasts for only five seconds or less, could be playing such an incredibly vital role in the physiology of life. Researchers were used to dealing with complex biochemical molecules with complex, polysyllabic names. NO wasn't like this; NO was simple. It just didn't make sense. Not since the 1921 discovery of insulin had there been such a revolutionary—and controversial—breakthrough in biochemical understanding.

In 1990, Drs. Moncada and E. Annie Higgs published *The 1990 Royal Society Symposium: Nitric Oxide from L-Arginine,* which revealed numerous new insights about cell function that were previously unimaginable and, for many scientists, still too fantastic to be believed. Dr. Moncada's introduction to the *Symposium* summed up the road to NO enlightenment:

> Several unrelated fields of research unknowingly paved the way to discovery that nitric oxide (NO), synthesized from L-arginine, plays a role as a regulator of cell function and communication. However, when the discovery was made, a number of scientists, used to dealing with endogenous substances such as peptides, amines or fatty acids, thought it impossible that such a molecule could play any biological role or even be synthesized by mammalian cells. Indeed in an era in which we are engineering and describing the roles of the most complex molecules, the simple combination of the two most common gases in the atmosphere seems a most unlikely biological mediator.[4]

As *The New York Times* reported in 1991, this incredulity was understandable: Nitric oxide "has escaped physiologists' attention until now because it survives in the body for a mere five seconds or so, and because it bears no resemblance to any known biological regulator."[5]

Difficult as it was to believe at first, the new revelations about ADNO have gone on to sweep the worlds of modern medical research in just a few short years, offering new potential for improving health in a broad spectrum of physiological systems. A standard medical textbook, *Cardiovascular Medicine*, already has an updated chapter on circulatory-system regulation wherein nitric oxide is cited as a *major aspect* of the factors known to regulate blood vessels.[6]

In 1992, NO was voted Molecule of the Year by *Science*, and consumer health publications like the *Harvard Health Letter* soon thereafter began running articles with titles like "Much Ado About NO" and "Say NO to Impotence?"

Serious research into ADNO exploded in the 1990s. Between 1980 and 1989, there were only a few dozen scientific publications on EDRF/nitric oxide. From 1990 on, research

Of Bulls, Bacteria, and Nitrites

In most male mammals with the exception of us primates, the penis when not in reproductive mode is safeguarded inside the body cavity thanks to the contraction of a special "retractor muscle." In order for a bull to become physically aroused, for example, this retractor muscle needs to get the signal to relax, followed by a similar signal to smooth-muscle tissues within the penis proper to relax as well. This second relaxation, which we primates do share in common with bulls, allows blood to cascade in, producing the hydraulic engorgement that is pumped-up male passion succinctly defined.

Until the discovery of ADNO, researchers had long believed that acetylcholine alone was the primary if not sole mediator of bullish passion. What they couldn't explain, however, was an odd physiological fact that bawdy bulls regularly excreted more nitrates than they took in from their feed. The discovery of ADNO finally explained why: To trigger erections, bulls were using L-arginine to make nitric oxide, which, in turn, was eventually eliminated from their bodies in nitrate form.

Such insights were among many that have helped researchers better understand the biochemistry of human erections, leading to new-generation drugs like the much-publicized Pfizer product Viagra (sildenafil citrate), the so-called anti-impotence pill that works by potentiating the effects of nitric oxide in the human penis.

Bulls, to be sure, weren't the only creatures excreting more nitrates than they ate. Researchers studying immune function found the same bizarre phenomenon in lab rats. Moreover, when rats in a completely germ-free environment were purposely infected with bacteria, their bodies produced an even greater urinary excretion of nitrates, showing that they were making more NO.

After much investigation, it turned out that rat immune-system cells were synthesizing NO from L-arginine, a process that eventually led to the elimination of nitrogen wastes as nitrates. But why immune cells were making ADNO remained a mystery for years, that is, until researchers discovered that they were using tiny "puffs" of the gas to actually kill invading bacteria.

Eventually, scientists would come to appreciate just how vital ADNO is to virtually all life functions, from the cardiovascular system and immune-system defense to nerve-cell communication and reproductive potency. Not only do all these systems depend on ADNO, but nature, in its wisdom, has given them the means to make it when it is needed.

began to escalate rapidly, and there were about 8,000 such publications by 1996. In 1997 alone, there were 5,000 such publications by the end of August.

Scientists have now also learned that there are at least three different variants of a special enzyme, called nitric oxide synthase, that instructs different parts of your body to make ADNO as needed. The endothelial cells have their own form of this enzyme (constitutive), which triggers ADNO-stimulated vessel relaxation, lowering blood pressure. Brain and nervous-system cells have a slightly different form of the enzyme, which may be the key to long-term memory. And different immune cell "soldiers" have yet another form (inducible) that allows them to produce NO to kill invaders.

The beauty of these different "isoforms" of nitric oxide synthase is that it allows different systems to make NO only when they need to, independent of the other systems.

As you will learn in coming chapters, the multitude of roles that ADNO plays in human health is truly astonishing. You will also see how different kinds of damage—by chronic hypertension, elevated serum cholesterol, atherosclerosis, oxygen free radicals, and many other causes—can impair your body's ability to make the ADNO it needs.

The good news is that you can give your body a major boost in replenishing ADNO by providing it with plenty of L-arginine from your diet and supplements. Indeed, some researchers are already saying that the discovery of ADNO—and the Arginine Solution it has spawned—is likely to become one of the most significant findings for health and wellness in the twenty-first century.

6

Supplemental Arginine
Loading Up on an Essential Raw Material

Tell me what you eat and I will tell you what you are.
—*Anthelme Brillat-Savarin, in* The Physiology of Taste, or Meditations
on Transcendental Gastronomy

Up until 1992, nitric oxide researchers had learned two things for certain: NO is essential to health, and L-arginine is the chief raw material the body uses to make it.

What was not so clear back then was whether giving patients additional L-arginine would translate into actual health benefits. Perhaps all the L-arginine that most of us need to meet our body's NO demands were the relatively modest quantities of it available in the average American burger-and-fries diet. If this proved true, then taking in extra L-arginine via supplements would likely be overkill.

But a pivotal 1992 clinical study conducted on heart patients in Japan found that when it comes to the benefits of ADNO, more is, indeed, more. In this study, patients were injected with thirty grams of L-arginine directly into their bloodstreams. This led to a rapid drop in blood pressure and a similarly rapid increase in the volume of blood pumped with each beat— dramatic and convincing cardiovascular benefits. Moreover, such treatment caused no serious side effects despite the fact that thirty grams represents *six times* the typical daily dietary intake of L-arginine.[1]

A host of other early clinical studies have time and again reconfirmed the benefits that follow intravenous delivery of arginine. Oftentimes a dose of arginine proves stunningly effective, triggering a normalization of blood pressure within mere minutes of an injection.

But why did the researchers choose to deliver the arginine by needle instead of by mouth? The reason they opted for injection over ingestion was that there were just too many uncertainties about how much oral arginine actually makes it into the bloodstream. It was easier to measure injected arginine precisely because it bypasses the digestive system altogether.

For obvious reasons, the average person hoping to benefit from ADNO doesn't want to have to inject him- or herself regularly to do so. As further research would eventually show, this has proven neither necessary nor desirable. Indeed, taking arginine orally via diet and/or supplements not only confers all of ADNO's health benefits, but also significantly prolongs its time of action.

Researchers have learned this thanks to several laboratory tests developed to measure nitric oxide concentrations in the blood. The first uses a special blood sensor that's usually inserted into a hand vein.[2] This sensor provides a highly accurate reading of arginine levels in the blood and the resultant changes in nitric oxide levels.[3] The chief disadvantage to this test is that it's invasive. Fortunately, other scientists have shown that you can also reliably estimate the NO in the blood by noninvasive techniques, i.e., by measuring either the quantity of NO a person exhales[4] or the amount of nitrates that shows up in urine.[5] Both these measures directly correlate with serum NO.

Thanks to these tests, scientists now know much more about how oral arginine makes its way into the body. They've learned, for instance, that some other amino acids, such as lysine, can interfere with arginine absorption. They've also learned that certain specialized immune cells in the gut called macrophages gobble up some arginine, further reducing the amount that enters the bloodstream. All in all, only about half of the arginine you ingest via food or supplements actually makes it to your circulatory system.

The good news is that the other half does gain entrance, and once it does so, it is available to work its magic throughout your body. Nor do you need take the same whopping doses given intravenously to begin seeing health benefits. Oral arginine doesn't work as quickly as injections of arginine, but it does appear to work as well, especially if taken regularly over time. Indeed, increasing your oral intake by only 50 to 100 percent of what you're already receiving from food can begin to impact your health positively in a few short weeks.

Dietary Arginine: Your Front-Line Defense

Long before nutritionists learned how to extract arginine from food, our only way to get sufficient ADNO was to eat products rich in it. The best sources have always been animal in origin: meat, poultry, fish, eggs, and dairy. Wild game is particularly high in arginine—there are over five grams of it in a single pound of venison or buffalo meat.

Arginine can also be found, though in much lower quantities, in certain vegetable sources, particularly wheat germ, legumes, nuts, and seeds. Fruits and vegetables, jam-packed as they are with other vital nutrients, contain almost no arginine.

If you're an average American, you are probably consuming about 100 grams of protein and 5.4 grams of arginine per day. If you're a heavy meat eater, chances are you're getting quite a bit more arginine to build muscles and help protect your heart, but also quite a bit more saturated fat and cholesterol to put your heart in need of help. If possible, try to stick to lean meats, "white meat" poultry, and especially fish—all great repositories for arginine but without the attendant heart-clogging baggage of fattier meats.

If, on the other hand, you're a vegetarian, especially one who eats no eggs or dairy products, you may well be getting inade-

Is Arginine "Essential"?

Nutritionists have long classified nutrients as either "essential" or "nonessential." This is a little misleading, because both categories are equally necessary for good health. The distinction simply has to do with the source of a given nutrient.

Essential nutrients are ones that your body can't produce naturally so it's essential you obtain them from foods or supplements. Nonessential nutrients, on the other hand, can be produced by your body, and for this reason the Nutrition Council suggests no RDA—recommended daily allowance—for them. Getting these nutrients from your diet is nonessential because your body can make what it needs.

The twenty-two amino acids humans require to stay alive abound in meat, eggs, dairy products, and other animal sources. You can also find them in various fruits, vegetables, and nuts, though getting sufficient quantities in the right combinations can be tricky. At least eight of the amino acids are inarguably essential, which is why pure vegetarians need to take such special pains to make sure a meatless diet doesn't cause a nutritional deficit.

Arginine falls into a gray area, with some nutritionists classifying it as essential, and others arguing that it's nonessential. It is true we can make arginine. What's controversial is whether we can make enough of it to meet our needs. A highly respected medical textbook, *Pathological Physiology*, by Drs. Sodeman and Sodeman, concludes that we often can't—and thus classifies arginine as essential.[7]

Semantics aside, arginine is the body's key source for nitrogen. It's not the only source; the nitrates in vegetables, for example, can help contribute the nitrogen necessary for nitric oxide synthesis. After reviewing the evidence, our own analysis has led us to believe that arginine *is* essential for many individuals, especially as they age. In the full bloom of youth, our cardiovascular and other bodily systems have not yet suffered the damage that so often comes with age. Most likely, we can meet all our arginine needs intrinsically at this point in life.

Not so in our latter years, when the cardiovascular system's need for ADNO is greater than ever, even as its ability to synthesize it has become compromised by years of heart-unhealthy habits. If you already suffer from atherosclerosis, hypertension, and the cavalcade of other chronic disorders—or if you fear you're heading in that direction—we believe that providing your body with extra ADNO is critical to your long-term health.

quate quantities of arginine. Others at risk for arginine deficiency include anyone on a fad diet that allows less than 1,000 calories total per day and those who stick to a high-carbohydrate, low-fat, and low-protein regimen.

To determine approximately how much arginine you're currently getting from the foods you eat, take a look at the accompanying chart. If your intake seems on the low side, or if you already suffer from cardiovascular problems such as hypertension that increase your body's need for arginine, it may be time to increase your daily intake.

Fortunately, there's an easy, safe, and inexpensive way to do this, one that doesn't require eating more animal products.

From "Power Formula" to Empowering Formula

Arginine is often combined in capsule form with another amino acid, L-ornithine, and marketed as a "power formula." The combination of these two amino acids, many bodybuilders believe, is particularly effective at stimulating the release of human growth hormone (HGH), which is so key to muscle development. (To be sure, too much HGH has, in recent years, been shown to fuel prostate growth and theoretically contribute to the risk of certain cancers. It's highly debatable whether any extra HGH released by relatively modest doses of L-arginine supplements has such effects, but if you currently suffer from prostate disease, please make sure to read more on any applicable caveats in Chapter 14.)

Arginine by itself is also easy to find. Indeed, as positive word of mouth continues to spread about this potent nutraceutical, it's becoming almost as readily available as vitamin C.

Powdered arginine is most often packaged in 500-milligram capsules. There are many distributors of arginine supplements; the products are available in most stores where health products are sold. See the appendix for a list of some of these distributors and their phone numbers.

How much is recommended? From our evaluation of medi-

FOOD	AMOUNT	CONTENT (g)
Wheat germ	1 cup	2.70
Granola	1 cup	.90
Oat flakes	1 cup	.60
Cheese	1 ounce	.20
Ricotta	1 cup	1.60
Cottage cheese	1 cup	1.40
Egg	1	.40
Whole milk	1 cup	.30
Chocolate	1 cup	.30
Yogurt	1 cup	.25
Pork	1 pound	5.24
Luncheon meat	1 pound	3.20
Sausage meat	1 pound	1.70
Chicken	1 pound	1.50
Turkey	1 pound	2.50
Duck	1 pound	2.20
Wild game	1 pound	5.20
Avocado	1	.10

TABLE 1

Many foods contain the amino acid arginine, but meats tend to be a particularly rich source for this vital nutrient. From E. R. Braverman and C. C. Pfeiffer, *The Healing Nutrients Within* (New Canaan, CT: Keats Publishing Inc., 1987), p. 169. Reprinted with permission.

cal research reports as well as the clinical benefits we've seen in our own patients, we suggest starting at a conservative dose of one gram taken three times per day. If this helps to lower your blood pressure, restore erectile function, and otherwise improve your health, we say wonderful—steady the course! But we often find that it is necessary to double this dose to the more commonly reported two grams taken three times a day to achieve full benefits.

Even at this "higher" level, arginine supplementation appears very safe. Nutritionists have also long considered arginine the least toxic of the amino acids, and its consumption, even in

	ESTIMATED INTAKE	
SOURCE	PROTEIN	ARGININE
	g/d	*mg/d*
Meat	30.3	2051
Poultry and fish	12.1	680
Dairy products	22.4	720
Eggs	6.3	405
Cereals	18.4	762
Other[1]	10.5	799
Total	100.0	5417

[1]The supply of arginine by other foods was calculated by assuming that the percentage contribution to this category was as follows: legumes, 35; nuts and seeds, 35; potatoes and sweet potatoes, 20; fruits, 5; and green and yellow vegetables, 5.

TABLE 2

Average per capita intake of protein and arginine in the United States by source. From W. J. Visek, "Arginine Needs, Physiological State and Usual Diets: A Reevaluation," in *Journal of Nutrition,* 116 (1986), pp. 36–46.

relatively huge quantities, seems to have very few adverse side effects.[6]

Numerous bodybuilders, for instance, have for years chronically consumed much greater quantities than our recommended dosage, and with no reported ill effects. Moreover, clinical trials at hospitals in the United States and abroad have repeatedly administered thirty to fifty grams a day of arginine safely to patients, again without reported problems.

Before starting on an arginine regimen, however, we urge you to discuss the matter with your physician to make sure there's nothing in your personal medical history to contraindicate such treatment. There are a few health conditions that may theoretically be exacerbated by arginine supplements (see Chapter 14). Though we believe the risk is extremely low at the dosages we endorse, prudence dictates a cautious approach if you do suffer from one of these disorders.

If your doctor does give you the green light, you can begin

arginine supplementation today as an adjunct to an overall integrated approach to good health. Eventually, a time-released formulation should become available, allowing you to take a single pill each morning. For now, however, you will need to take the supplement morning, noon, and night—a little aggravating, perhaps, but a small price to pay for the benefits you'll reap.

It's best to take each dose with some carbohydrates to prevent possible stomach upset. Avoid eating protein at the same time you take the supplement because this may interfere with the digestive absorption of arginine.

7

Pressure Drop
The Natural Way to Lower High Blood Pressure

Hold out! Relief is coming!

—*William Tecumseh Sherman*

"When my family physician told me that I had high blood pressure, I could hardly believe it. I'm only forty-three years old, and I've always taken excellent care of my health. I rarely get sick, my diet is low in saturated fat and high in fruits and vegetables, and if anything I'm a little underweight thanks to a daily regimen of running. In fact, I'm signed up to run my third consecutive New York Marathon. How could I *possibly* have high blood pressure? I thought only smokers and overweight couch potatoes had to worry about hypertension."

—Harold M., 43*

"After my divorce, I went through six months of chronic fatigue, pounding headaches, and an almost constant craving for salty foods. I thought these symptoms were just physical manifestations of the stress my marital breakup was causing me. I felt lousy but figured I'd eventually muddle through. Then one

*The stories of "Harold M." and others appearing in this book are meant to be illustrative of common health concerns. Some of the case studies have been based on composites of different patients.

night, I went over to a local health clinic to pick up a nurse friend whose shift was letting out. She took one look at me: the bags under my eyes, the weight I'd gained, the stressed-out wreck I'd become. She sat me down and said, 'Barb, I'd like to check your blood pressure.' When the reading came back 210/ 110, I just about lost it. My friend said I was stroke material and needed to see a doctor immediately. I was in shock—two years ago, my blood pressure was perfectly normal."

—Barbara T., 48

"To get my blood pressure under control, my doctor urged me to exercise, lose weight, cut back on alcohol, and try to handle stress better. Easy for him to say. My job as a salesman involves constant traveling, schmoozing clients at expensive restaurants, pressure to produce from the home office—not exactly conducive to any of the doctor's lifestyle recommendations. My idea of handling stress is a couple of double martinis at the end of a sixteen-hour day. Needless to say, the next time I saw my physician, my blood pressure was even higher than before, and he put me on medication. The good news is the pills are keeping my hypertension in check. The bad news is the stuff kills my sex life. My wife doesn't know this, but I stopped taking them a few days each week so we can still enjoy some kind of intimacy."

—Frank S., 51

Harold, Barbara, and Frank are just three of the 58 million Americans who suffer from hypertension, aka high blood pressure. Untold others are heading along in their footsteps. Often referred to as the "silent killer" because the disorder so rarely announces itself with any warning signs, hypertension is one of the leading causes of illness, disability, and death in the United States. Left untreated, chronic elevation of blood pressure nearly triples your risk of all the major circulatory disorders, from heart failure to peripheral artery disease. Hypertension does this by hurting you in a myriad of ways. It accelerates the hardening of your arteries, damages your heart by enlarging one or more of its chambers, increases the risk of blood clots that can trigger heart attacks and strokes, and can even lead to a rupture of a blood vessel in your brain, causing a so-called hemorrhagic stroke.

Perhaps you've already been diagnosed with hypertension yourself. Perhaps your blood pressure is now normal but a history of the condition runs in your family. Or maybe you've just watched a disturbing trend over the years, as your numbers have slowly climbed from low normal in your twenties and thirties, to normal in your forties, to borderline in your fifties, to who knows what in the future.

Unfortunately, the likelihood of further escalation has been well documented. The renowned Framingham Heart Study, for example, followed several generations of residents in the town of Framingham, Massachusetts, over forty years, taking detailed cardiovascular health assessments on each person every two years. One of the more intriguing findings: Fully two-thirds of participants who started out with normal blood pressure readings in their thirties had developed some degree of hypertension by their sixties.[1]

Other studies have shown that African Americans are particularly vulnerable to hypertension. Researchers for the National Institutes of Health in Washington, D.C., recently found that this vulnerability seems to be due to a reduced sensitivity of blood vessels to nitric oxide.[2]

Women of all races tend to enter adulthood with lower blood pressure than men, but by middle age they tend to catch up, and they often exceed blood-pressure levels in males of the same age.

Regardless of your own circumstances today, chances are you'd like to take whatever prudent steps you can to keep your blood pressure under control now and in the future, especially if you can do so with a minimum of dependence on medicines that may have serious side effects.

As many patients have begun to discover, there is now an effective, safe, natural treatment—the Arginine Solution—that can in most cases help control pressure without simultaneously causing depression, sexual dysfunction, or other adverse effects.

In Harold's case, six grams daily of supplemental arginine should allow him to normalize his blood pressure within seven weeks without the necessity of further medication. For Barb and Frank, prescription medication would usually still be necessary, but arginine supplements should allow each to reduce significantly the amount of prescription medicine they require. Encouraged, both have started to work more diligently on embracing healthier lifestyles: losing weight, exercising regularly, drinking less alcohol, cutting back on salt, and increasing their daily intake of vitamins, antioxidants, and foods rich in calcium, potassium, and magnesium.

The bottom line: Both now have an excellent prognosis, and may eventually be able to go off prescription drugs altogether.

How It Works: The Direct ADNO Link to Blood Pressure

On one level, blood pressure is relatively easy to understand. You've got a given volume of blood being pumped through a series of pipes forming a closed system. The force against the walls of these pipes is your blood pressure. When your heart contracts, forcing blood forward, the pressure temporarily goes up. This is known as the systolic blood pressure, i.e., the maximum force, measured in milligrams of mercury, placed on your artery walls. When your heart relaxes between beats, the pressure momentarily drops to its baseline, your so-called diastolic blood pressure.

Note: An easy way to keep these terms straight is to remember that systolic, the higher number, starts with an *s*, whereas diastolic, the lower number, starts with a *d*. In the alphabet, *s* is "higher" than *d*.

The pipes in question bear little resemblance to the inflexible copper tubing that carries water throughout your house. Rather, they're living tissues that are truly a marvel of dynamic flexibility. With each contraction of the powerful left chamber of your heart, oxygen-rich blood is propelled forward into your aorta, the body's largest artery. From here, the blood flow di-

Salt Sensitivity and ADNO

The fact that hypertension can sometimes run in families has led research-ers to search for genetic influences in the disorder. One of the most likely of these has to do with how your body handles salt.

In most people, consuming as much as three teaspoons of salt per day re-sults in no discernible changes in blood pressure. Physicians say that these indi-viduals are salt-resistant—i.e., their bodies somehow resist any adverse effects from excess sodium.

But a sizable percentage of other individuals fall into the "salt sensitive" category. For these folks, even seemingly insignificant increases in sodium in-take can lead to a quick rise in blood pressure. The most likely reason: The sodium in salt results in water retention, which increases blood volume. The more blood volume in a closed system, the greater the pressure on the pipes. Sodium also triggers the production of hormones that can directly or indirectly cause blood pressure to rise.

Doctors still don't completely understand the exact biomechanisms that allow some people to handle salt easily while others react to it by increasing their blood pressure. Perhaps the latter was an adaptive trait at one point in human evolution, a safeguard against water loss in desert environments. But as beneficial as salt sensitivity may have been for those in arid regions, the modern world has converted the erstwhile advantage into a handicap. Sodium is ubiq-uitous in the American diet, an impossible-to-avoid component of salty snack foods, to be sure, but also lurking covertly in everything from flavorings such as malt extract and MSG to over-the-counter medicines such as antihistamines and laxatives.

If you're one of the lucky ones who is not salt-sensitive, you can eat your pretzels with impunity. If, on the other hand, your blood pressure reacts to the faintest whiff of sodium, you will need to take special care to eliminate as much of it as possible from your diet.

Though both groups can also benefit from ADNO supplements, emerging evidence suggests these benefits will occur more rapidly for the salt-sensitive population.

In a recent study published in the *American Journal of Physiology*, researchers fed a high-salt diet to lab rats genetically bred to resist the effects of sodium on blood pressure. The rats met the increased dietary "salt challenge" by making ad-ditional nitric oxide, which protected them from any increases in blood pressure.

The researchers then fed the same high-salt diet to salt-sensitive rats. These animals, alas, proved incapable of making extra nitric oxide in response. Their blood pressure skyrocketed and their kidney function deteriorated. Could anything other than sodium reduction normalize these problems? To find out, the researchers continued feeding the salt-sensitive rats a high-sodium diet but supplemented this with arginine. Very quickly, both blood pressure and kidney function returned to normal—compelling evidence for ADNO's ability to preserve circulatory health.[10]

In another study published in *Hypertension,* researchers wanted to determine what role ADNO plays in normal dogs, i.e., animals not bred to be genetically salt-sensitive. As expected, these dogs met an increased salt challenge by urinating more frequently and excreting more sodium in their urine. The bottom line: Blood pressure remained steady. The researchers then administered a drug that temporarily inhibits nitric oxide formation from arginine. The dogs' blood pressure suddenly soared—testament to the fact that ADNO is one of the chief means by which dogs counter a salt challenge.[11]

Evidence gleaned from rats and dogs is encouraging, but do the same principles apply to people? Tantalizing evidence suggests that the answer is yes. Dr. Michael D. Brown and colleagues at the University of Michigan reported in *Circulation* the results of a study of fifteen middle-aged, slightly overweight patients suffering from high blood pressure. They found that humans, like lab animals, respond differently to a dietary salt challenge depending on whether they are salt-sensitive or salt-resistant.[12] Hypertensive individuals whose ability to create NO from arginine is unimpaired can generally lower blood pressure simply by cutting down on salt. But in those whose ADNO production capacity has been compromised, perhaps by atherosclerosis or other damage to the endothelium, restricting salt does little to normalize blood pressure.

In either case, adding supplemental arginine may be just the ticket your body needs to set things right.

vides into other large arteries, which, in turn, branch off into progressively smaller arteries and, eventually, the tiny arterioles, which give way to even tinier capillaries. The function of the arterial system, from the aorta to arterioles to capillaries, is the expeditious transportation of blood to every organ and tissue in your body.

To be sure, there are many times when some parts of your body require more oxygen and nutrients than others. If you're

Classification of BP in Adults Aged 18 Years or Older*

BP RANGE, MM HG	CATEGORY†
DBP	
<85	Normal BP
85–89	High-normal BP
90–104	Mild hypertension
105–114	Moderate hypertension
≥115	Severe hypertension
SBP, when DBP	
<90 mm Hg	
<140	Normal BP
140–159	Borderline isolated systolic hypertension
≥160	Isolated systolic hypertension

*Classification based on the average of two or more readings on two or more occasions. BP indicates blood pressure; DBP, diastolic blood pressure; and SBP, systolic blood pressure.

†A classification of borderline isolated systolic hypertension (SBP, 140 to 159 mm Hg) or isolated systolic hypertension (SBP, ≥160 mm Hg) takes precedence over high-normal BP (DBP, 85 to 89 mm Hg) when both occur in the same person. High-normal BP (DBP, 85 to 89 mm Hg) takes precedence over a classification of normal BP (SBP, <140 mm Hg) when both occur in the same person.

Follow-up Criteria for Initial BP Measurement for Adults Aged 18 Years or Older*

BP RANGE, MM HG	RECOMMENDED FOLLOW-UP
DBP	
<85	Recheck within 2 y
85–89	Recheck within 1 y
90–104	Confirm within 2 mo
105–114	Evaluate or refer promptly to source of care within 2 wk
≥115	Evaluate or refer immediately to source of care
SBP, when DBP	
<90 mm Hg	
<140	Recheck within 2 y
140–199	Confirm within 2 mo
≥200	Evaluate or refer promptly to source of care within 2 wk

*BP indicates blood pressure; DBP, diastolic blood pressure; and SBP, systolic blood pressure. If recommendations for follow-up of DBP and SBP are different, the shorter recommended time for recheck and referral should take precedence.

TABLE 3

From the 1988 Report of the Joint National Committee on Detection, Evaluation, and Treatment of High Blood Pressure, in *Archives of Internal Medicine*, 148 (1988), pp. 1023–1038.

Upper or Lower: Is One Number More Important?

For decades, the conventional wisdom in medical circles has been that elevated diastolic blood pressure (the lower number) is more worrisome than elevated systolic pressure (the higher number). But is the conventional wisdom correct?

It turns out that there is little compelling data supporting this supposition. If anything, elevated systolic pressure may actually be *more* dangerous to heart health than elevated diastolic pressure. In men of all ages who were followed in the Framingham Heart Study, for instance, the incidence of heart disease, stroke, cardiac failure, and peripheral artery disease was substantially greater for those with elevated systolic (and normal diastolic) readings than for those with elevated diastolic (and normal systolic) readings.

Though correlations are far from simplistic, and the presence of other factors such as a history of heart attack can confound risk ratios, the basic lesson seems clear: If your systolic blood pressure is elevated, seek treatment even if your diastolic readings are normal.

Just as you would use a scale to monitor your progress if you were intent on losing weight, it is desirable to monitor your blood pressure if you are taking arginine supplements to reduce it. Any conventional self-inflating instrument obtainable at your local drug store will do the job. It has not been reported that arginine supplementation lowers blood pressure in persons in whom that pressure is normal. Nevertheless, to be on the safe side, we recommend that you monitor your blood pressure regularly to avoid any possibility of developing low blood pressure. Should you develop low blood pressure, it would be wise to cut back on the arginine supplementation and confer with your doctor about what dosage may be appropriate for you.

jogging, for example, your skeletal muscles, particularly the large muscle mass in your legs, require plenty of oxygen and energy sources to fuel contractions. On the other hand, after a heavy meal, it's your digestive system that needs extra attention—one reason, perhaps, for the collective national nap following Thanksgiving dinner engorgement. If you've ever suffered cold hands and feet on a frigid winter day, you also know firsthand how well your body automatically shunts blood from your extremities to guarantee that your vital core temperature remains at a healthy 98.6°F for as long as possible.

But how does your circulatory system accomplish this amazingly complex logistical task, i.e., preferentially delivering blood to exactly where it's most needed at any given time? It does this, in large part, by selectively dilating the "pipes" that carry blood to high-demand regions while constricting those that supply regions that are lower on the priority list. Doctors refer to these two complementary mechanisms as vasodilation (opening up some arteries so more blood can flow through them) and vasoconstriction (narrowing other arteries so less blood goes through them). Your arterial system, in turn, accomplishes this opening and narrowing via the action of smooth-muscle rings that wrap around the arterial "pipes" themselves. Think of a flexible garden hose surrounded by an Ace bandage. Tighten the bandage and less fluid gets through. Loosen the bandage and more can advance.

A variety of chemical signals can tell your smooth-muscle "Ace bandages" to relax or contract. Alcohol, for instance, can temporarily relax smooth muscle and open up vessels throughout your body, which is one reason why a stiff drink on a cold day can make your hands and feet feel warm, even as it increases your risk of hypothermia by impairing the adaptive shunting of blood to your body core.

Men who get drunk and then have trouble attaining an erection might wonder why this would be so. If alcohol opens blood vessels, wouldn't this mean more blood flow to the penis, ergo an erection? The problem is that alcohol opens vessels indiscriminately. It's akin to turning on all the spigots in your house, then wondering why the water pressure in your shower is so pathetic.

Operating properly, however, the smooth-muscle action is anything but indiscriminate. It is, instead, a miraculous example of biochemical orchestration, with the principal conductor of this orchestra being—you guessed it—nitric oxide derived from arginine. Certain blood-borne substances such as norepinephrine definitely play a role in causing arterial blood vessels to

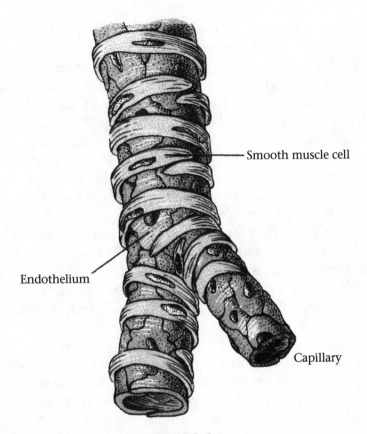

Smooth muscle cell

Endothelium

Capillary

FIGURE 2

Arterioles are like living pipes that carry oxygen and other nutrients to the body's tissues. Smooth muscle cells ring these vessels, expanding or constricting blood flow as needed. The principal regulator for smooth muscle relaxation: ADNO, or nitric oxide, made from arginine by endothelial cells. From Gerald Tortora and Nicholas Anagnostakos, *Principles of Anatomy and Physiology*, 4th edition. Copyright © 1983 by Biological Sciences Textbooks Inc., A&P Text, and Ella Sparta, Inc. Reprinted by permission of Addison Wesley Educational Publishers.

constrict, whereas other substances, such as acetylcholine, play a role in their relaxation. We do not mean to overly simplify this process, because it is so bewilderingly complex that researchers are still at a loss to explain in detail how it happens.

What researchers do now know is that ADNO is integral to most if not all of these processes. This means that the arginine-derived nitric oxide created by the endothelial cells lining your arteries is now known to be the *principal blood pressure regulator* of the body.

Once produced and released by the endothelium, nitric oxide causes the arterial smooth muscles making up the vessel walls to relax, loosening the "Ace bandage" effect, enlarging the interior diameter of the artery, and ultimately letting more blood flow through.

It has only recently been discovered that damage from the standard coronary heart-disease risk factors, from hypertension to high cholesterol, impairs the ability of your endothelium to produce nitric oxide when and where it is needed.

The good news is that highly compelling evidence now suggests that arginine supplements can help restore that balance. Arginine can both resurrect endothelial cells that have already been damaged and provide these and undamaged cells with an increased supply of the building blocks needed to make nitric oxide. The bottom line: Even if your natural capacity for vasodilatation has already been damaged, ADNO can still help lower your blood pressure and restore health to your circulatory system. And if your arteries aren't damaged, the Arginine Solution promises to help keep them that way for years to come.

At this point, you may be wondering how oxygen and nutrients can ultimately penetrate their way through the muscular artery walls to nourish the body's cells. The answer is, they don't. The arterial system is designed to transport blood; the actual delivery takes place via capillaries, tiny blood vessels that are only a single cell thick and lack any smooth-muscle rings. Oxygen and soluble nutrients pass through the capillary walls to your cells, which, in turn, surrender carbon dioxide and metabolic wastes back into the capillaries. Then the circulatory system begins its return trip via tiny veins that give way to progressively larger veins that eventually carry blood to the kidneys for waste excretion and to the lungs where CO_2 is exhaled and new oxygen is picked up. Then it's back to the heart for the next round trip.

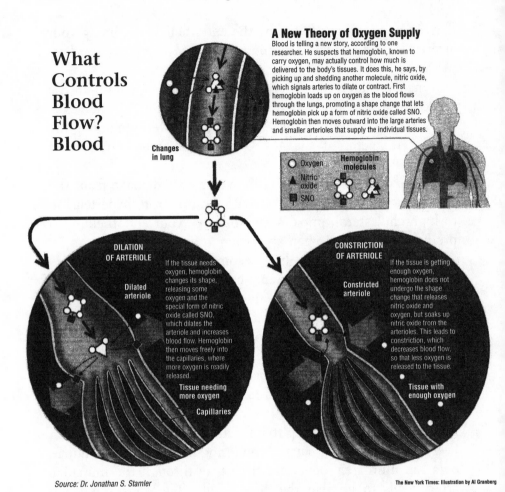

What Controls Blood Flow? Blood

A New Theory of Oxygen Supply

Blood is telling a new story, according to one researcher. He suspects that hemoglobin, known to carry oxygen, may actually control how much is delivered to the body's tissues. It does this, he says, by picking up and shedding another molecule, nitric oxide, which signals arteries to dilate or contract. First hemoglobin loads up on oxygen as the blood flows through the lungs, promoting a shape change that lets hemoglobin pick up a form of nitric oxide called SNO. Hemoglobin then moves outward into the large arteries and smaller arterioles that supply the individual tissues.

Changes in lung

Oxygen
Nitric oxide
SNO
Hemoglobin molecules

DILATION OF ARTERIOLE

Dilated arteriole

If the tissue needs oxygen, hemoglobin changes its shape, releasing some oxygen and the special form of nitric oxide called SNO, which dilates the arteriole and increases blood flow. Hemoglobin then moves freely into the capillaries, where more oxygen is readily released.

Tissue needing more oxygen

Capillaries

CONSTRICTION OF ARTERIOLE

Constricted arteriole

If the tissue is getting enough oxygen, hemoglobin does not undergo the shape change that releases nitric oxide and oxygen, but soaks up nitric oxide from the arterioles. This leads to constriction, which decreases blood flow, so that less oxygen is released to the tissue.

Tissue with enough oxygen

Source: Dr. Jonathan S. Stamler   The New York Times: Illustration by Al Granberg

FIGURE 3

A new theory of oxygen supply. Copyright © 1996 by the New York Times Co. Reprinted with permission.

Unlike arterial vessels, which have encircling smooth muscles that can increase or decrease blood flow to targeted tissues as needed, veins have no such smooth-muscle rings. The reason is straightforward: Once blood has become oxygen-depleted and waste-laden, it needs to be filtered and replenished. It doesn't matter where in the body the blood happened to surrender its oxygen and pick up waste materials—all of it has the same priority for reprocessing in the kidneys and lungs.

Because veins are essentially passive conduits, blood pressure is largely regulated by the smaller vessels of the arterial system, which doctors call the "resistance vasculature." To be sure, there are definitely disease processes that can hurt your veins, from so-called varicose veins where pooled blood, in essence, gets stuck, to painful blood clots that can migrate through the circulatory system and cause obstructions. Still, when it comes to regulating blood pressure, your arterial system—and its absolute dependence on ADNO—is clearly the most important factor.

Giving Your Vessels a Break with ADNO

As any savvy business manager knows, a staff expected to work for too long at full throttle without breaks is a staff headed for burnout or a breakdown. Thus it is with your resistance vasculature. Give your arteries a breather and they'll pay you back with reliable, steadfast service. But subject them to chronic high-pressure overloads and they'll eventually deteriorate.

As we've already seen, ADNO powerfully relaxes the smooth-muscle arterial rings that, when dilated, decrease blood pressure. The Arginine Solution boosts ADNO, and in so doing, it provides additional raw materials that enable your remaining healthy endothelial cells to undertake the same job that a fuller complement of them can handle. Finally, there is growing evidence that supplemental arginine taken regularly over time can begin to heal damaged endothelial cells and return them to their pre-injury level of functioning. The bottom line: Supplemental arginine, when taken in concert with a healthy approach to living, can help keep your blood pressure where your vessels need it to be.

The alternative, to be sure, is to let your blood pressure remain chronically high—and watch your blood vessels pay the price. Indeed, the increased sheer stress on your artery walls leaves them more vulnerable to a variety of damage, everything from vessel-clogging plaque formation to ruptures of this plaque that can trigger blood clots and obstruction.

This damage, in turn, can further impair the endothelium's ability to produce NO, which means your arteries will stay even more constricted and your blood pressure will spike even higher. This, of course, only guarantees worse vessel damage, a vicious downward spiral whisking you toward premature disability and early death.

What the Journals Say

The treatment of high blood pressure with ADNO clearly makes theoretical sense given the dual benefits of relaxing arteries and, as you will see in Chapter 10, inhibiting blood clots. But does it really work in real patients?

Hundreds of research articles, as well as our own clinical practice, suggest that the answer for many patients is a resounding yes! At the risk of inducing "study shock," here's a short sampling of recent research:

- In a clinical study reported in *Journal of Cardiovascular Pharmacology*, five patients with high blood pressure were given intravenous arginine. They had an average blood pressure of 154.5/95 mm Hg before getting arginine, but shortly afterwards, their systolic blood pressure dropped an average of nearly 30 mm Hg and the diastolic blood pressure decreased an average of 22 mm Hg.[3]
- In another clinical trial published in *The Lancet*, hypertensive men ranging in age from thirty-five to sixty-five volunteered to withdraw from blood pressure medication for up to one week. Each morning, they were given intravenous arginine one hour before breakfast. This caused a rapid decrease in both systolic and diastolic blood pressure in these patients, an effect that lasted for twenty minutes. No side effects other than dry mouth were reported.[4]
- Other researchers have wondered whether arginine supplements taken orally might have a more long-lasting

benefit than arginine via injections. A recent study, which was first presented in November 1997 at the American Heart Association's 70th Scientific Session and later published in *Circulation,* looked at patients ranging in age between thirty and seventy and suffering mild to moderate hypertension (i.e., blood pressure greater than 160/90 mm Hg). The researchers found that an oral arginine supplement of 2,000 milligrams per day worked to lower their blood pressure significantly.[5]

- Numerous other studies now corroborate this finding that oral ADNO can successfully reduce elevated blood pressure. One recent study that appeared in the *Journal of the American College of Cardiology* in 1998 looked at fourteen patients in Italy newly diagnosed with borderline high blood pressure. The researchers found that it took only two grams a day of L-arginine administered orally for a week to trigger nearly twenty point drops in systolic blood pressure—a fact they credited to L-arginine's ability to improve endothelial function.[6]

Don't Fear the White Coat

Diagnosing high blood pressure can be tricky. More than a fifth of all patients with "in-the-doctor's-office" readings higher than 140/90 actually have normal blood pressure when readings are taken at home. The long-term consequence of so-called white coat hypertension is not yet known, but at least one five-year study has found no increased cardiovascular risk to patients who simply get nervous in a medical setting. Because of this, multiple out-of-the-office readings are probably a better gauge of your true blood pressure.

If normal readings at home do confirm that your hypertension is of the "white coat" variety, you probably don't need prescription drug therapy to treat it. Instead, consider making any lifestyle changes that are needed, including exercise, a better diet, and arginine supplements.

The Thorn in the Rose

If you've been diagnosed with high blood pressure, chances are your doctor has already advocated a healthy lifestyle as the first line of defense. But if a wholesome diet, regular exercise, weight loss, stress management, and other common-sense strategies fail to bring your blood pressure under control, you've probably been told that medication will ultimately become necessary.

We believe that for many patients suffering borderline to moderate high blood pressure,[7] supplemental arginine can serve as a catalyst to open blood vessels and optimize the power of healthy lifestyle choices. Even if you still need to take prescription drugs, arginine can reduce the amount of medication you depend on, and may eventually allow you to go off prescriptions altogether. This is important because high-blood-pressure medicines, as effective as they can be, can also have serious attendant side effects.

Since many of you may already be taking these drugs alone or in combination, here is a short primer on the most commonly prescribed classes currently available:

Diuretics or "Water Pills"

These medicines, which have been used for nearly forty years, are typically the first choice for many patients. They work by causing your kidneys to excrete more salt and water, which, in turn, reduces the fluid volume of your blood. It's analogous to a water balloon filled almost to the bursting point. If you can remove some of the water, the balloon is that much less likely to burst. Common diuretics include thiazides (Hydrodiuril), furosemide (Lasix), and spironolactone (Aldactone).

Beta-Blockers

You're no doubt familiar with what a jolt of adrenaline can do. The body's natural turbocharger triggers heart-pounding, wide-eyed, fight-or-flight power, allowing one parent reportedly to lift a Volkswagen to save an imperiled child. It's a nice power to have, at least in reserve, but for those of you who suffer from high blood pressure, an adrenaline rush is the last thing you need. Adrenergic blockers block the effect of these overstimulating hormones, kiboshing the pounding heart, soaring blood pressure, sweating, shaking, and other physical manifestations of stress. Older-generation drugs like beta-blockers work on nerve sites throughout the body. Indeed, some are so effective for masking the external symptoms of anxiety that they've developed something of a cult following among concert musicians and public speakers as a cure for stage fright. Taking a beta-blocker pill before a performance helps guarantee that the performance won't be wrecked by tremulous limbs or a quavering voice.

Newer-generation adrenergic blockers are more selective, working mainly on target receptors in the heart and blood vessels. Many of these drugs also signal the kidneys to filter out and remove certain hormones, such as renin, from the blood, hormones that would otherwise lead to constricted blood vessels. Common examples of beta-blocking drugs include metoprolol (Lopressor), propranolol (Inderal), and atenolol (Tenormin).

Calcium Channel Blockers

These relatively new drugs work by reducing the entry of calcium into the smooth-muscle cells that encircle our arteries and arterioles. Smooth muscles require calcium to contract, so the less calcium that makes its way inside the cell, the less contraction that takes place, allowing vessels to remain relaxed and dilated. Examples of calcium channel blockers include verapamil (Calan), nifedipine (Procardia), and diltiazem (Cardizem).

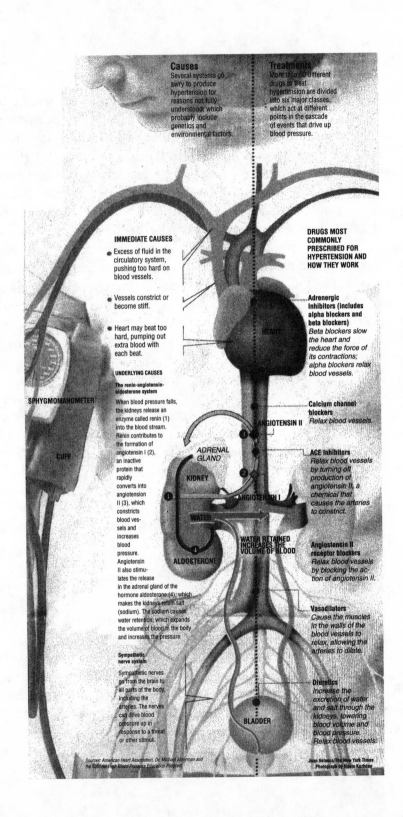

Causes
Several systems go
awry to produce
hypertension for
reasons not fully
understood, which
probably include
genetics and
environmental factors.

Treatments
More than 60 different
drugs to treat
hypertension are divided
into six major classes,
which act at different
points in the cascade
of events that drive up
blood pressure.

IMMEDIATE CAUSES

- Excess of fluid in the circulatory system, pushing too hard on blood vessels.

- Vessels constrict or become stiff.

- Heart may beat too hard, pumping out extra blood with each beat.

UNDERLYING CAUSES

The renin-angiotensin-aldosterone system

When blood pressure falls, the kidneys release an enzyme called renin (1) into the blood stream. Renin contributes to the formation of angiotensin I (2), an inactive protein that rapidly converts into angiotension II (3), which constricts blood vessels and increases blood pressure. Angiotensin II also stimulates the release in the adrenal gland of the hormone aldosterone (4), which makes the kidneys retain salt (sodium). The sodium causes water retention, which expands the volume of blood in the body and increases the pressure.

Sympathetic nerve system

Sympathetic nerves go from the brain to all parts of the body, including the arteries. The nerves can drive blood pressure up in response to a threat or other stimuli.

SPHYGMOMANOMETER

CUFF

HEART

ANGIOTENSIN II

ADRENAL GLAND

KIDNEY

ANGIOTENSIN I

WATER

WATER RETAINED INCREASES THE VOLUME OF BLOOD

ALDOSTERONE

BLADDER

DRUGS MOST COMMONLY PRESCRIBED FOR HYPERTENSION AND HOW THEY WORK

Adrenergic Inhibitors (includes alpha blockers and beta blockers)
Beta blockers slow the heart and reduce the force of its contractions; alpha blockers relax blood vessels.

Calcium channel blockers
Relax blood vessels.

ACE Inhibitors
Relax blood vessels by turning off production of angiotensin II, a chemical that causes the arteries to constrict.

Angiotensin II receptor blockers
Relax blood vessels by blocking the action of angiotensin II.

Vasodilators
Cause the muscles in the walls of the blood vessels to relax, allowing the arteries to dilate.

Diuretics
Increase the excretion of water and salt through the kidneys, lowering blood volume and blood pressure. Relax blood vessels.

Sources: American Heart Association, Dr. Michael Alderman and the National High Blood Pressure Education Program.

Juan Velasco/The New York Times
Photograph by Naum Kazhdan

ACE Inhibitors

The human body is a complex marvel of biochemical chain reactions, fail-safe mechanisms, redundant systems, and feedback loops, the result of which is a high degree of control over physiological functions. Put a little more simply, the body usually provides "more than one way to skin a cat." The regulation of blood pressure is no exception. It turns out that one of the signals for blood-vessel constriction is a hormone known as angiotensin II. A naturally occurring enzyme called ACE (for angiotensin-converting enzyme) causes the body to make angiotensin II from angiotensin I, which itself is made from the kidney hormone renin. When researchers finally figured all this out, they developed drugs that inhibit ACE, which keeps angiotensin II levels low, which means that vessels get less stimulus to constrict. ACE inhibitors include enalapril (Vasotec), captopril (Capoten), and lisinopril (Zestril).

As effective as they are, all these medicines have the potential for creating new problems in the patients who take them. *The New England Journal of Medicine* cautioned almost fifteen years ago that beta-blockers and diuretics, for example, can cause thinking impairment and medical complications, including some that may lead to blindness, inflammatory joint disease, *increased risk of coronary heart disease,* and impotence.[8]

These are not rare footnotes, either. In a survey of patients, the British Medical Research Council reported that nearly one in six men and one in eight women on beta-blockers and/or

---

FIGURE 4
(facing page) **Principal causes of high blood pressure and conventional medical tactics to lower it. Although ADNO has received a great deal of attention for its ability to lower blood pressure rapidly and safely, it is still not included in the list of treatments for that condition.** Copyright © 1998 by the New York Times Co. Reprinted with permission.

diuretics for hypertension withdrew from treatment due to adverse effects. These included headaches, nausea, dizziness, lethargy, constipation, skin disorders, impaired glucose tolerance, and shortness of breath.[9] Like a vaudevillian chest of drawers, when you use these medicines to solve one problem, often another will pop up to clout you on the knees.

For male patients, one of the most common, and pernicious, of these new problems is impotence. Indeed, the British Medical Research Council found that men who remained on the drug regimen for two years had a nearly one in four chance of becoming impotent. Both diuretics and beta-blockers were shown to cause this impotence, though the effect was more pronounced with diuretics.

What about the newer-generation drugs, medications for which the hype is matched only by the price tag? It turns out that calcium channel blockers, especially the short-acting forms, may actually increase, not decrease, the mortality of patients who have already suffered a heart attack.

Potential side effects and uncertainties notwithstanding, the damage caused by untreated hypertension can be devastating. If your doctor has prescribed medication, you should definitely take it. But you should also let your doctor know if the drugs trigger problems, for often a change in dose or a switch to another class of medication can help you control your blood pressure without ruining the quality of your life.

Perhaps most importantly of all, approach any drug treatment not as a substitute for but as an adjunct to an overall healthy approach to living. From weight loss to exercise to arginine supplementation, the best way to gain control of your blood pressure is first to gain control of your life.

As part of a plan to lower your blood pressure, we also recommend that you monitor it regularly. Any of the commonly available automatic blood-pressure-monitoring devices, such as those found at your local drugstore, will do the job. Be sure to calibrate it with your physician for accuracy. Monitoring will help you see progress in lowering elevated pressure. It will also tell you when to cut back on the dosage once it normalizes, thus avoiding the possibility of hypotension, or blood pressure that's too low.

Blood pressure is regulated by a variety of complex biochemical mechanisms, including blood-borne substances, nitric oxide, and other molecules that variously constrict or relax arteries, speed up your heart rate, and/or cause your platelets to clump. The first-line defense against hypertension includes embracing a healthy lifestyle—i.e., eating well-balanced meals and losing weight, exercising, avoiding cigarette smoking and excessive alcohol consumption, reducing sodium if you are "salt sensitive," and reducing stress.

If these measures aren't sufficient to normalize your blood pressure, you should definitely talk to your doctor about medications to prevent the "silent killer" from adding you to its victim list.

In addition to—and sometimes instead of—prescription pharmaceuticals, oral arginine supplementation has been shown to be a safe and effective way for you to get your blood pressure down if it's elevated, or to keep it down if it's still within normal limits. You and your doctor will need to keep in mind that it can take several weeks for arginine to effect a measurable drop in blood pressure. We've had success treating patients with a starter dosage of one gram taken three times a day, eventually increasing this to two grams three times a day if the lower dose fails to produce enough of a drop.

In cases where arginine alone may not be potent enough to return high blood pressure to a safer range, taking arginine along with certain prescription medications could still have a significant complementary effect. It may allow you to get by on less medication than you might otherwise need—and therefore suffer fewer or milder side effects. The bottom line: Arginine supplements provide your cardiovascular system with one of the raw materials it needs to function optimally. With or without additional medicine, it's a good way to take care of your blood vessels and your heart. Arginine supplements are available from a number of distributors such as Real Health Laboratories and may be found in most stores and pharmacies where health products are sold. See the appendix for a list of some of these distributors.

8

Of ADNO, CAD, and Athero
Heart Health and Plaque Prevention

This sickness doth infect the very lifeblood of our enterprise.
—*William Shakespeare:* Henry IV

"On a hot afternoon last summer, I found myself experiencing some hard-to-describe chest pains—not terrible, crushing pains, just a distinctly uncomfortable tightness. Despite having had a good night's sleep, I also felt extremely fatigued and short of breath. My wife told me I needed to be checked out by our family doctor immediately. I told her it could wait, that my symptoms were no big deal. Thank God she didn't buy into my denial.

"When we arrived at the doctor's office, he spent about five minutes checking me over before concluding that I needed to go to the emergency room for more tests. There, a cardiologist determined that one of my coronary arteries was over 90 percent blocked by atherosclerotic plaque. He called my condition coronary artery disease, or CAD, and said it needed attention as soon as possible. That same day I agreed to have a procedure called balloon angioplasty.

"To enlarge the vessel opening, the surgeon snaked a tiny deflated 'balloon' up through my leg artery to the site of the plaque. Then he temporarily inflated the balloon to expand my

artery from the inside. Afterwards, he put in a vascular stent—
basically a small tube device—to help keep my now opened artery from renarrowing.

"A couple of days after this surgery, I was sent home from
the hospital feeling pretty good physically but not so great psychologically. For years I'd suffered both high blood pressure and
high cholesterol, plus heart disease definitely runs in my family.
Somehow, I'd convinced myself that none of these risks would
ever apply to my own chances of getting heart disease. My doctor told me I'd come very close to suffering a full-fledged heart
attack that could have killed me. And he said that if I don't
change my lifestyle and take the medication he's prescribed, it
probably will happen eventually."

—Peter N., 55

"I feel like I've been battling high cholesterol my entire adult
life. I first discovered I had a problem when I was twenty-two
and the doctor found that my total cholesterol was 252. My
'good' HDL cholesterol was forty-two, not great but not horrible, either. So I went on this strict diet she recommended, and
three months later I got retested. On the plus side, my total
cholesterol had dropped to 228. On the negative side, my good
HDL had dropped to 36.

"My doctor explained that you want the ratio of total cholesterol divided by HDL to be under 4. She said that though my
overall cholesterol level had dropped, my HDL fraction had
dropped proportionately faster, so the net effect was that my
ratio had actually risen from 6 to 6.3. Depending on what
school of cardiology you subscribe to, the result of all my dietary
self-denial was that my risk of heart disease was now actually
higher than before!

"I continued on the low-fat diet for another three months,
only to see the same trend continue. My total cholesterol de-
clined to 212, but my protective HDL remained virtually constant at 35. Truth be told, I was sick of avoiding all the foods
I'd liked my whole life. So I just said to hell with it and went

back to eating and drinking whatever I wanted. I just made up my mind that it wasn't worth worrying about it.

"A couple of years later, I had to get my cholesterol tested again because I was applying for life insurance. The results: Overall cholesterol had skyrocketed to 309. But my HDL had also risen to 48. My ratio was now at 6.4, as bad as it had ever been.

"So far, I have no signs of heart disease. I'm an exercise nut, and I can run the mile almost as fast at forty-five as I could in high school. I've asked several doctors what I should do, and I've gotten the same answer. They want to put me on these new-generation cholesterol-lowering drugs like Zocor [simvastatin], Mevacor [lovastatin], or Pravachol [pravastatin]. Never mind that my health insurance is terrible, and that at two dollars or more a pill, the cost of these medicines would all be coming out of my own pocket."

—Scott T., 45

Heart disease: Five million Americans have it, 500,000 die from it each year, and countless others worry obsessively about getting it. Though too much worry can be counterproductive—stress, after all, may up your odds of developing the condition—it only makes sense to take prudent action now to avoid becoming a mortality statistic in the future. Even if you've already been diagnosed with heart disease, it's never too late to start doing something about it. Don't mope, don't throw your arms up in surrender: Fight back, and take control of your health. And as you will soon see, the Arginine Solution can play an integral part in an all-out, take-no-prisoners assault on this most ubiquitous of killers.

The first step is to educate yourself about the causes of a wounded heart—and the remedies for it. Start with the fact that there are many different forms of heart disease, from problems in electrical signaling, to inflammation caused by an infection like rheumatic fever, to congenital heart-valve deformities. But two specific preventable kinds of heart disease account for the vast majority of cases.

The one you are probably most familiar with is obstructive coronary artery disease, or CAD, a condition characterized by coronary vessel blockages that reduce the blood reaching the heart proper. In this chapter, we will discuss how atherosclerosis, or hardening of the arteries by cholesterol-laden plaque, plays a major role not only in coronary artery disease, but also in the most common form of stroke, peripheral artery disease, and high blood pressure itself.

A second form, so-called hypertensive heart disease, has received much less press, but it can be just as devastating. It occurs when the heart itself actually changes in form and function as a result of chronic untreated high blood pressure. When these changes become severe enough, the heart strains to pump sufficient blood to meet the body's demand, a condition also known as congestive heart failure. If you have been diagnosed with this form of heart problem, feel free to skip ahead to Chapter 9, where we discuss the condition's causes—and possible remedies, including the Arginine Solution.

The Framingham Study[1] and other large-scale epidemiological studies have found that your chances of developing both these types of heart disease depend in large measure on whether or not you have various risk factors. Some of these risks you can't do anything about. For instance, you can't change your gender—and men *are* statistically at much greater risk for developing early heart disease than women. After menopause, however, the estrogen that once protected the feminine heart plummets, and older women quickly catch up to older men in their rate of heart disease. Age and a family history of heart disease are other risk factors you can't do anything about. As much as many of us might wish it, we can neither stop the clock nor retroactively pick our parents.

Fortunately, there are many other "modifiable" risk factors that can be even more potent influences on your heart health. And with these, you absolutely can do something about them:

- If you're a smoker, you can stop.
- If you're obese, you can shed some pounds.

Where There's Smoke, There's Heart Disease

T he more researchers discover about the multiple and vital roles nitric oxide plays in human health, the more apparent it becomes how important it is to keep our levels of NO high. Supplemental arginine is one great way to do this.

But another great method, if you're currently a smoker, is to quit this habit *now!* To be sure, slides of autopsied lungs from dead smokers—organs blackened by tar and shredded by emphysema—show one direct result of tobacco's villainy. But what can be just as ruinous, though admittedly harder to visualize, is the effect smoking has on your body's ability to make nitric oxide.

In a study published in *The American Journal of Respiratory and Critical Care Medicine,* investigators recently compared the nitric oxide exhaled by forty-one smokers with "healthy" lungs (i.e., no emphysema, lung cancer, or other diagnosable disease *yet*) with the nitric oxide exhaled by a comparable group of nonsmokers. This kind of lung measurement gives a good indication of how much, or how little, NO the body is producing. The bottom line: Smokers were producing less than half the NO of nonsmokers.[14]

If you think such results afflict only heavy smokers, think again. Another study found that smoking *one* cigarette decreased exhaled nitric oxide by 33 percent.

A report in 1996 in *Circulation* concluded that smoking damages the endothelium of blood vessels and sets the stage for atherosclerosis. One likely mechanism, the authors suggested, was impaired nitric oxide formation.[15]

On the plus side, another researcher found that nitric oxide levels begin to return to normal within fifteen minutes of the last cigarette smoked. Chain-smokers, alas, will never see this. But for those who can cut back and eventually quit smoking altogether, healthy levels of NO—like the light at the end of the tunnel—await to work their physiological magic on your healing cardiovasculature.

- If you're sedentary, you can incorporate regular exercise into your daily life.
- If you're constantly stressed out, you can learn—and regularly practice—proven stress-management techniques like meditation, biofeedback, and yoga.

- If you have an unhealthy lipid profile—i.e., high "bad" cholesterol and triglycerides, low "good" cholesterol—you can improve your diet by decreasing saturated fat and "trans fats" (those that have been partly or entirely "hydrogenated") and increasing fiber, particularly the soluble form found in oat bran, psyllium, and other sources.
- If you have a high level of the protein homocysteine in your blood, you can take vitamins B_6 and B_{12} and folic acid to bring it down.
- If you suffer from diabetes, you can help keep your blood sugar under control.
- And finally, if your blood pressure is chronically elevated, you can take a variety of measures to depressurize. These measures include all of the above—*plus* the three to six grams of supplemental arginine recommended in the previous chapter.

To be sure, not all these ways of fighting back against heart diseases will be easy to adopt. If nicotine were not so powerfully addictive, for example, there certainly wouldn't still be millions of hooked smokers wishing they could quit. For many other people, losing weight can be even harder than kicking cigarettes; studies show that most dieters will eventually gain back hard-lost pounds.

But as difficult as it can be to live a healthier lifestyle, it's certainly not impossible. Remind yourself that every small step helps. Moreover, one of the effective measures, the Arginine Solution, is exceptionally simple. All you need to do is remember to take a supplement three times a day.

In Chapter 7, we showed you how ADNO can keep your endothelium healthy and your blood pressure in check. Now take a moment to see why this is also such a beneficial gift you can bestow on your heart.

And the Winner Is . . .

In 1997, Dr. Rainer H. Boger and his colleagues at the Hanover Medical School in Germany decided to perform a side-by-side comparison of oral L-arginine versus lovastatin in the lowering of cholesterol. Lovastatin (trade name: Mevacor) was the first approved medication in the so-called statin class, potent cholesterol-lowering chemicals being increasingly recommended as a treatment for all elevated levels of cholesterol.

Indeed, by the time of Dr. Boger's experiment, many physicians had come to accept the fact that the statins were the new gold standard against which all other cholesterol-lowering medicines must be measured. Few expected L-arginine to come close to lovastatin's effectiveness.

An animal "model" often used to study atherosclerosis is the rabbit because its blood vessels, like ours, respond to a high-fat diet by forming deposits of cholesterol plaque inside the artery walls. Dr. Boger and his colleagues fed their test animals a 1 percent cholesterol diet for four weeks, then followed this with a 0.5 percent cholesterol diet for twelve more weeks. This may not sound like all that much cholesterol, but it's easily enough to promote significant plaque formation in rabbits over a relatively short time period.

Though all the rabbits received the same food, they didn't all get the same beverage. Here Boger divided them into three groups. The first group received plain drinking water. The second drank water laced with lovastatin. And the third got water containing dissolved L-arginine.

As expected, the rabbits who received no treatment showed significant atherosclerotic plaque in vital arteries, including the carotids that supply the brain and the aorta that supplies the body. Moreover, their artery walls had noticeably thickened, narrowing the inside diameter of these vessels. Finally, these "plain water" rabbits also suffered an impaired ability to make nitric oxide from ADNO. The bottom line: These test subjects were well on their way to obstructive artery disease.

Also as expected, the group of rabbits receiving lovastatin-laced water along with their high-cholesterol diet did enjoy some significant protection. Specifically, these animals showed less plaque formation in their brain and heart arteries, less thickening in vessel walls, and less degradation of ADNO production.

What was surprising, however, was the effectiveness of L-arginine at fostering the same changes lovastatin had brought about. Indeed, oral L-arginine didn't just measure up to the gold standard—it *exceeded* it.

The study, which was published in the August 1997 issue of *Circulation,* the official journal of the American Heart Association, concluded that "lovastatin had a weaker inhibitory effect on carotid plaque formation and aortic artery intimal [vessel wall] thickening than L-arginine."[2]

Equally provocative was the researchers' finding that L-arginine seemed to inhibit so-called oxygen free radicals, the much-publicized biochemical bogeymen that wreak such havoc on living tissues unless they're neutralized by antioxidants. Lovastatin, on the other hand, not only didn't inhibit oxygen free radicals, it even seemed to *energize* them. The study adds a definite spot of tarnish to the miracle drug's halo, intimating that even as it works to cure heart disease with its right hand, a statin drug may be tacitly encouraging other kinds of damage with its left hand.

When you factor in recent research suggesting that the high-priced statin drugs can promote side effects in people that range from cognitive impairment to cancer,[3] the Arginine Solution emerges as an even more attractive option for controlling cholesterol and its health consequences.

What's Up, Doc?

At this point, you may be saying "Okay, so maybe arginine works on rabbits—but I'm not a rabbit! What about people?"

For obvious reasons, doctors can't intentionally set out to induce atherosclerosis in people just to see if arginine can help them. What researchers can do is to look at patients who already suffer high cholesterol and atherosclerosis and see what effect, if any, arginine has on their condition. Consider just three of the studies published in top medical journals that have addressed precisely this question:

- *The New England Journal of Medicine* reported in 1993 that patients with advanced atherosclerosis of the lower limbs as well as hypertension and elevated serum cholesterol were given intravenous arginine on each of seven consecutive days. The infusion rapidly lowered plasma cholesterol levels for up to twelve hours. The authors concluded that the observed effect was due to the conversion of arginine to nitric oxide.[4]
- *The Lancet* also recently reported a clinical effort at the Utrecht University Hospital in the Netherlands to reverse cardiovascular disease in patients diagnosed with elevated cholesterol. Patients with advanced vascular disease were taken off drugs prescribed to lower their serum cholesterol levels for a period of two weeks. After that time, and compared to a control group, they already showed a significant impairment of the ability of the endothelium to produce nitric oxide and dilate the small arterial blood vessels. The drug treatment was reinstituted and the difference between the patients and the control group disappeared after three months. Then the patients were taken off drugs again, and both they and the control subjects were given an intravenous infusion of arginine. Arginine infusion had about the same effect in the patient group as did the cholesterol-lowering drugs.[5]
- In a study conducted at Sinai Hospital in Baltimore and published in the *Journal of Perenteral & Enteral Nutrition*, healthy elderly patients were given seventeen grams of oral arginine per day for two weeks. This decreases total cholesterol and LDL without also reducing the "good" HDL cholesterol. The bottom line: The patients enjoyed a significant improvement in their lipid profile. And despite the relatively high dosage, no adverse side effects were observed.[6]

These and a growing body of other human and animal studies continue to strengthen the case for ADNO as a potent cholesterol-lowering supplement. But please do not misunderstand our intentions in relating this information. If your doctor has already prescribed medication, *don't* unilaterally stop taking it and make the switch to arginine. *Do,* however, discuss the growing evidence for arginine with your health-care provider to see if adding it as a complement to your current treatment makes sense in your situation.

We believe that a conservative dosage of three to six grams of oral arginine daily will help lower your cholesterol and, as you will see later in this chapter, prevent its conversion into a particularly dangerous "oxidized" form that contributes so substantially to plaque. In some cases, taking oral arginine regularly may let you eventually lower the statin dose and perhaps go off it altogether.

And if your cholesterol is not yet elevated to the point where you need medication, the Arginine Solution can help you to stay that way. Earlier in this book, we revealed the way ADNO can treat or prevent high blood pressure. In the next chapter we describe the deleterious heart changes untreated hypertension can cause over the years. In this chapter, we will look at ADNO's beneficial effects on another key element in cardiovascular diseases: atherosclerosis, commonly known as hardening of the arteries.

If this deleterious process occurs in the slender but vital arteries that supply your heart muscles with oxygen and nutrients, it can lead to the aptly named CAD, or coronary artery disease, which greatly ups your risk of a heart attack. If the carotid arteries supplying your brain harden, you become vulnerable to a brain attack, that is, the most common kind of stroke. Though these two atherosclerosis-related catastrophes are the most feared by many patients, hardened arteries elsewhere in the body can lead to other physical problems with sometimes devastating consequences, as someone who suffers the pain of peripheral artery disease—the result of hardening of the arteries that supply the calves, thighs, hips, and feet—can tell you.

Though all these conditions occur in different parts of the

body, they all have one causative factor in common: the narrowing of vital arterial vessels by atherosclerotic plaques.

The White Plague

The bubonic plague of medieval times killed off one out of every four people in Europe. During the death throes, a victim's body often turned a telltale purple color due to respiratory failure, a symptom that earned this virulent bacterial infection a grisly sobriquet: the Black Death.

But before you let yourself feel too much smug relief that mankind has at last escaped its plague years, consider this: The White Plague of our own modern world is responsible not for 25 percent of human deaths in the United States and Western Europe—it's responsible for over 45 percent!

To be sure, the culprit is not *Yersinia pestis* transmitted by fleas that bit rats and then people. Rather, it's a natural white crystalline compound found in the fats and oils of animals, a chemical the body requires to make cell membranes, vitamin D, and many key hormones. Indeed, so critical is cholesterol to human health that the liver is programmed to produce over 50 percent of our daily level—more than we get from the foods we eat.

Unfortunately, it's all too easy to get much more cholesterol than we need from a diet rich in dairy products and meats. In some people, there's so much surplus that cholesterol-rich bile in the gallbladder gets crystallized into the agonizing deposits known as gallstones.

Not that you need to take in an abundance of dietary cholesterol to suffer from high cholesterol levels. Certain kinds of fats that remain solid at room temperature—like the saturated fat in butter or the "trans" vegetable fats that have been partially or wholly "hydrogenated" for use in snack foods—can cause the liver to manufacture more cholesterol. Indeed, it's possible to eat a diet virtually devoid of any cholesterol and still have high blood levels of it because of the liver's production.

You might have an image of cholesterol as so many fatty blobs, microscopic versions of the tallow droplets that appear in refrigerated roast beef juice. Though the blood of people with extraordinarily high cholesterol does look almost oily, serum cholesterol is not generally visible to the naked eye. In fact, researchers have discovered that certain proteins serve as carriers for cholesterol in the blood. The two most significant of these proteins are low-density lipoproteins, or LDL; and high-density lipoproteins, or HDL.

Depending on which of these proteins that cholesterol is bound to, it can either promote hardening of the arteries or work to prevent it. In a sense, you can think of the "H" in HDL as standing for "heroic" because it carries cholesterol out of your system, and the "L" in LDL for "lethal" because it can contribute to the formation of plaque that narrows and hardens your arteries.

We all have both kinds of cholesterol, but some people have a better "lipid profile" than others, which means they have more of the good relative to the bad. You want to keep your total cholesterol (the main component of which is LDL) as low as possible while keeping your HDL as high as possible. Indeed, if you divide the total amount by the HDL, the resulting ratio should be 4 or lower. Most physicians now realize this ratio is actually more important in deterring cardiovascular risk than total cholesterol alone.

For example, a person with a "desirable" level of 180 milligrams (mg.) of total cholesterol per deciliter (dl.) of blood could actually be at high risk if his or her HDL measured only 30 mg./dl. But another person with the same 180 total reading could be at very low risk if his or her HDL measured, say, 60 mg./dl. The first person's ratio is a whopping 6; the second's is a very heart-healthy 3.

All this sounds fine on the drawing board, of course, and your doctor has no doubt already told you the variety of strategies for boosting the heroic while lowering the lethal. Quit smoking, exercise more, drink alcohol moderately—these can all help raise HDL. Lose weight and avoid eating foods high in saturated fats, trans fats, and cholesterol—reductions here can all help lower LDL.

Alas, these techniques don't always work for everyone. The liver of genetically susceptible individuals seem stubbornly committed to countering any dietary reduction in cholesterol by simply manufacturing more of it. There's also the seductiveness of our fat-abundant fast-food culture that makes it hard to sustain even the best intentions for very long. Indeed, even those who have been "scared straight" by a first heart attack can find it difficult to adhere to a low-fat diet year after self-deprived year.

Boosting HDL, on the other hand, can be even more difficult than lowering LDL. The much-touted use of aerobic exercise, for instance, doesn't work for nearly half of all people with low HDL, no matter how much they exercise. Drinking alcohol, though arguably more reliable in increasing HDL, has its obvious health drawbacks. A goblet of red wine at every meal may let the French survive their pâté de foie gras, croissants, and buttercream desserts, but in the United States, the "French paradox" seems more likely to translate into increased traffic fatalities, domestic violence, and cirrhosis. Ours is a culture more prone to excess than cultured moderation.

Fortunately, the complex processes that ultimately lead to artery-occluding plaque offer numerous avenues for intervention. As you will see, ADNO can powerfully and positively affect plaque formation at several of these different stages. But to see how, first take a minute to understand better how atherosclerosis develops—and the spiraling damage it can cause.

From Streaks to Stenosis

The first stage of atherosclerosis occurs when fatty streaks called atheromas begin to appear on the walls of arterial vessels. As indicated earlier in Chapter 4, the presence of these fatty streaks has been documented by autopsy in soldiers as young as eighteen felled in combat. If you eat a typical American diet, chances are excellent you have at least some of these fatty streaks already in your own circulatory system.

If you were to look at the components of an atheroma under a microscope, you'd find primarily a ragtag collection of immune-system cells, from white blood cells to a special type of macrophage, or cellular "gobbler," which surrounds oxidized LDL and, in the process, changes into what physiologists call a foam cell. You can almost think of foam cells as tiny cholesterol garbage bags, but instead of safely discarding the refuse outside the body, they end up getting stuffed just beneath the surface of the vessel wall. It's sort of the biochemical equivalent of sweeping dirt under the rug.

Though fatty streaks may appear at random sites in your arteries, the earliest deposits tend to accumulate in places where the blood flow is particularly turbulent and prone to changes in velocity, especially where an artery narrows. Anyone who has driven on a busy highway system knows where the "turbulent" sections are most likely to occur—not on straightaways but rather on curvy stretches of road or intersections where new roads merge or branch off. These are the sites where accidents are most likely to happen. These are the same places in your circulatory highway where plaque deposition is most likely to begin.

The initial plaque builds, layer by layer, thanks in large part to another type of blood cell, your platelets. Platelet function, and the effect of ADNO in regulating this, will be discussed in much more detail in the following chapter. For now, suffice it to say that your platelets perceive an atheroma as an injury to your blood vessel. When they arrive on the scene, they quickly trigger a meshwork of collagen and fibrin that fixes the layer of cholesterol garbage bags in place. Arterial smooth-muscle cells begin to grow abnormally around this. As macrophages gobble up and deposit more LDL over the years, the layers of accumulating plaque grow thicker and more solid.

During the end stages of plaque formation, a once-fatty streak begins to take on calcium and harden. The core of the plaque now contains dead and abnormal cells that have leaked out cholesterol crystals like so many rotting garbage bags. The plaque also contains numerous elastic and collagen fibers as well as deposits of the aptly named GAG (glycosaminoglycans).

Such a grotesque mass is called a thrombosis, and it can become so thick that it encroaches into the artery channel, or lumen. Doctors refer to this occlusion as stenosis, from a Greek word meaning "to narrow." An estimated 400,000 patients in the United States each year undergo so-called balloon angioplasty, the same procedure that Peter N. had, to reopen such narrowed arteries from the inside. Unfortunately, in many cases, the arteries "re-stenose" as the plaque formation sags back or rebuilds.

To be sure, an artery that has become severely narrowed by atherosclerosis is dangerous for multiple reasons. In the next chapter, you'll see how a rupture in this plaque can trigger blood clots that totally choke down blood flow. When this happens in your brain, you can suffer a stroke; in your heart, a heart attack. These are well-publicized health catastrophes, but no part of your body is immune. When blood ceases to flow to a limb, for instance, there's always a chance that you can develop gangrene and you may require an amputation.

But atherosclerosis also wreaks much of its havoc in more subtle ways. It can prematurely age and disable us. It can impair memory in the middle-aged, and foster a form of senile dementia in the elderly. It can impair proper circulation to any organ and cause peripheral artery disease and high blood pressure. When blood flow to the sex organs is impaired, atherosclerosis can produce impotence. As we'll discuss in the next chapter, even a modest amount of hardening of the arteries may actually be the leading cause of hypertension. All these seemingly different disorders have the same common cause: hardening of different arteries by calcified cholesterol plaque.

The good news is you don't have to suffer from any of these problems. Even if you've already been diagnosed, you can begin to reverse the damage done and return to good health. The Arginine Solution, along with a healthy lifestyle, can play an invaluable role in helping you reduce cholesterol and rejuvenate your blood vessels. Read on to find out why.

Stopping the Radicals

Leave a stick of butter out of the refrigerator long enough, and it eventually turns rancid due to a chemical reaction known as oxidation. A similar oxidative reaction occurs, albeit more slowly, when iron rusts and, more quickly, when combustible materials catch fire.

Unfortunately, oxidation is not confined to butter, iron, and bonfires. It also goes on constantly inside living tissues. During metabolic reactions, highly reactive molecules known as oxygen free radicals can initiate a kind of chemical chain reaction that, left unchecked, can damage cell membranes, alter DNA, convert harmless fats into killers, and trigger a rogues' gallery of disorders from cancer to cataracts. Indeed, one of the leading theories for why we age and eventually die is the cumulative impact of oxidative damage to our cells and tissues.

It's impossible to avoid free radicals altogether, though minimizing your exposure to radiation, toxic chemicals, pollutants, and even charbroiled meat is only prudent since all of these can spawn a surfeit of free radicals. The use of antioxidant nutraceuticals—such as vitamin E, vitamin C, and now arginine—can help eliminate the free radicals that do make it into your tissues.

For those interested in protecting their arteries from plaque, antioxidant treatment is quickly emerging as one of the most critical aspects of self-care. Why? It now appears that LDL is most likely to result in plaque deposition only when it has been oxidized. The reason: Unoxidized LDL doesn't exert much attraction to the fat-gobbling macrophages. Oxidized LDL, on the other hand, proves an irresistibly delicious target. And once a macrophage zeroes in and envelops the "rancid" oxidized form of LDL, it turns into a foam cell, attaches to the inside of an artery wall, and adds yet another tiny piece to the developing atherosclerotic brickwork.

So, you might now be wondering, why not just eliminate all the free radicals from your body? There are two main reasons why this is both impossible and undesirable. For one thing, free radicals arise as a natural by-product of numerous metabolic reactions we need to live. Some of the key examples of these unstable "oxygen species" include superoxide (O_2), hydroxyl (HO), hydrogen peroxide (H_2O_2), peroxynitrite (ONOO), and—surprise, surprise!—nitric oxide (NO) itself.

As you will see in Chapter 12, the human body actually uses NO and other free radicals as potent immune-system weapons to kill off invading infectious disease and to counter cancer. Even if we could prevent free radical formation, it would hardly be in our best interests to do so.

Antioxidant ADNO

But this doesn't mean we can't control free radicals when an excess threatens to cause more harm than good. Undoubtedly, you've already witnessed the tremendous publicity given to antioxidant vitamins, key "good guy" scavengers like vitamin E, vitamin C, and the family of carotenes and bioflavonoids, which roam about the bloodstream donating electrons and thus neutralizing free radicals. Though much research continues on how, where, and to what extent these antioxidants work to prevent disease, the evidence now is overwhelming that preventing LDL from becoming oxidized is one of the keys to preventing atherosclerotic plaque.

Indeed, many cardiologists have begun routinely recommending daily vitamin E for just this purpose.[7] One reason it appears so beneficial: Unlike water-soluble vitamin C, vitamin E is fat-soluble, which means it can more easily attack the lipid molecules circulating in our blood.

But as heralded as vitamin E has been in recent years as a potent preventer of LDL oxidation, there is now another supplement with equal if not greater promise: L-arginine. Indeed, researchers from the Medical College of Wisconsin recently found that ADNO can be as effective at preventing LDL oxidation as vitamin E, but at a much lower relative dose.[8]

But this isn't all it can do for you. Researchers at Stanford recently found that ADNO supplementation actually reduces the tendency for immune system cells to attach to vessel walls, even when serum cholesterol is high and free radicals abundant.[9] These same conditions, when ADNO is in short supply, are practically a guarantee of significant plaque deposition.

A few of the other intriguing findings from recent research include:

- To see if arginine could help restore function to vessels damaged by plaque, researchers at the College of Medicine at Texas A & M University looked at the coronary blood vessels in two groups of living pigs. The first group had been fed a healthy diet and still had clean arteries. The second had been fed a high-fat diet and as a consequence had developed significant atherosclerosis. The researchers inserted tiny arterial lines into the pigs' coronary arteries to record vessel changes in response to increased blood flow. In the healthy group, such an increase prompted the arteries to undergo a natural dilation. But in the pigs whose heart arteries had hardened with plaque, there was no such "flow-mediated" expansion.[10] This is a particularly significant finding for humans, as well, because we too depend on these flow-mediated blood-vessel adjustments to stay healthy. The good news for the pigs: An infusion of arginine rapidly restored normal function to heart arteries whose endothelial layers had been damaged by plaque.

- You don't have to be an atherosclerotic lab animal to benefit from arginine. A study in the journal *Circulation* revealed that long-term oral arginine supplementation in people with elevated cholesterol and atherosclerosis actually reduced pathological increases in the thickness of plaque-lined vessel walls.[11]

- Another *Circulation* study found that oral arginine supplements of 7,000 milligrams, taken in divided doses, three times a day for as few as three days in a row, improved blood-vessel relaxation in young men with elevated serum cholesterol and coronary artery disease.[12]
- The 1997 supplement to the *Journal of the American College of Cardiology* included a study involving certain heart patients at the Mayo Clinic. Researchers found that 8.4 grams given to these patients three times a day significantly enhanced coronary artery blood flow.[13]
- Yet another clinical study published in *Circulation* showed that a total of 7 grams per day improved blood flow in men, aged fifty-five to seventy-seven, with elevated serum cholesterol and early coronary artery disease.

Oral Versus Intravenous Administration

As we discussed briefly in Chapter 6, arginine can be administered directly into a patient's bloodstream via an injection, or delivered orally through a dietary supplement. Many clinical studies report giving patients arginine by injection. The reason: When a person suffers advanced disease, the intravenous route guarantees that arginine can go to work rapidly to reduce symptoms. This doesn't mean, however, that swallowing arginine in supplement form is less effective. On the contrary: Oral arginine taken regularly has time and again proven its ability to lower cholesterol, prevent LDL oxidation by free radicals, restore endothelial function, normalize blood-vessel dilation, reduce platelet stickiness, and generally tune up your cardiovascular system.

Compared with injection, oral arginine may take a little longer to get to work. But it more than makes up for this in terms of a steady, long-lived effect. Taking three to six grams daily, divided into three equal doses over the course of the day, will help ensure that your body always has the ADNO it needs to keep your system operating at its best.

* * *

High levels of cholesterol in the blood have long been linked to atherosclerosis, heart disease, and other circulatory disorders. The process by which plaque becomes deposited inside artery walls is complex. It begins when LDL cholesterol is oxidized by free radicals. This makes it an irresistible target for immune system cells called macrophages that engulf the LDL, convert into foam cells, and seep into the walls of blood vessels.

Over time, this results in endothelial cells becoming more and more separated from their arterial blood supply. As endothelial function declines, blood pressure increases, which in turn hastens further plaque deposition. As these pathological processes repeat themselves over and over again, a fatty streak progressively evolves into full-fledged calcified plaque. The latter contains a mix of dead and abnormal cells, crystallized cholesterol, and other cellular debris. Blood cells called platelets rush to "repair" the damage—but only succeed in exacerbating blockages.

A variety of studies now indicate that regular doses of oral arginine may help prevent and potentially even reverse atherosclerosis via two distinct biochemical mechanisms. First, it can lower serum cholesterol without also lowering the good HDL cholesterol fraction. Second, it can act as a potent antioxidant to prevent the formation of the dangerous oxidized form of LDL.

9

When Hearts under Pressure Swell
The ADNO Rx for Preventing Disaster

> So the heart is the beginning of life, the Sun of the
> Microcosm . . . by whose virtue and pulsation, the blood is
> mov'd, perfected . . . and is defended from corruption.
> —*William Harvey*

"My father had high blood pressure for as long as I can remember. I know that as an African American I stand a better-than-average chance of getting it myself. A couple of years ago, my dad started to suffer some heart problems, and the doctor told us it was probably because his high blood pressure had gone untreated for so long that it put stress on his heart muscle and caused it to beat irregularly. He's on medication now, which seems to be helping. But I'd sure like to avoid following in his footsteps if I can. So far my own blood pressure is *usually* normal, but I want to keep it from creeping up."

—Brian B., 31

"I've always told myself that because I'm a woman, my risk of heart disease is modest at best. But since enduring menopause, I've read more and more articles suggesting that I can be just as much at risk for a heart attack as men my age. I'm fifty-five and work as a medical receptionist in a group medical practice, so you'd think I'd take all the cardiovascular health warnings seriously. I *do* try to keep my weight under control and rarely drink more than a glass of wine a day. But I'm definitely not as active as I should be—some days, my only exercise consists of walking to and from my car. My big vice is cigarettes. I smoke almost a pack a day, more when I'm really feeling stressed. The last time I got it checked, my blood pressue was borderline high.

"In recent months, I've started to suffer some on-again, off-again symptoms that have got me concerned. I'll get these occasional slight chest pains—I can't really even pinpoint their location. Sometimes it doesn't even feel like pain at all but just a tightness sensation and a feeling of breathlessness. These symptoms can fade away for weeks at a time. But then they're back. They can strike when I'm active, or when I'm resting, and sometimes when all the office phones are ringing off the hook at once. I get frazzled trying to page different doctors when all the callers are in a hurry and snapping at me. In fact, just thinking about this aspect of my job makes my chest tighten. I try to rationalize it as just a normal stress reaction. But I can't help but wonder if I'm fooling myself."

—Stephanie M., 55

"My mother smoked for years, and she drank at least three or four mixed drinks almost every night. Her doctor first diagnosed her with hypertension when she was in her early fifties and he put her on pills for it. Unfortunately, the pills triggered a serious bout with depression, so she went off medication after only a few months. When she was sixty-six, her doctors discovered the lung cancer that would lead to her death in less than a month. Her actual cause of death, however, wasn't cancer but congestive heart failure. The doctors told us her heart just couldn't carry the load anymore.

"I'm forty-five now, and I swim on a masters' swim team three or four times every week. In fact, I came in first in the 100-yard butterfly in the regional meet this past spring. I've never smoked, I eat a good diet, and I meditate to help inoculate myself against the stress of my job as an art teacher. My own blood pressure has been low normal for years, but at my last checkup, it was a little elevated. My doctor thought it was probably only 'white coat hypertension'—just a case of nerves when they were doing the test. But I also get heart palpitations now and then, and I end up focusing my attention on my heart. Believe me, the heart is an organ I'd just as soon *not* notice. My doctor told me not to worry about this stuff, but the fact is I *am* worried. My mom's death was not an easy one, and I'm determined to do everything I can to keep my own cardiovascular system healthy. It's almost as if I feel I owe it to my mom and myself to benefit from her example. I'm just not sure what more I can do."

—John R., 45

In Chapters 7 and 8, we examined the ways untreated high blood pressure and atherosclerosis can impair your health, sometimes with devastating consequences that include heart attacks, strokes, and peripheral artery disease. These conditions rarely exist in a vacuum. High blood pressure, for instance, can escalate the rate of atherosclerosis, and atherosclerosis can cause blood pressue to soar. Indeed, hardening of the arteries is fast emerging as one of the single most important causes of hypertension.

But the damage doesn't stop here. If you've ever sprained an ankle and had to limp around for a week or two, you've probably noticed that your other leg may begin to hurt because of the additional strain it suffers while compensating for the original injury. A similar kind of thing can happen to your heart as well, when it's forced to adapt to the heightened workloads placed on it by hypertension and atherosclerosis. In a very real sense, your heart is simply doing its best under arduous circumstances. But subject it for too long to this added burden and the "adaptations" the heart is forced to make can end up ruining its ability to function.

Of Athletes and Broken Hearts

You're probably well aware that a "normal" blood pressure reading is generally considered 120mm Hg for systolic pressure over

Stopping Snakes from Chasing Each Other's Tail

H igh blood pressure can be caused by numerous physiological problems, but one of the more intriguing possible villains is early atherosclerosis—so early, in fact, that it can't yet be diagnosed by conventional noninvasive tests. In fact, by the time the average person reaches early middle age, the arteries are about half "cholesterol-ized."

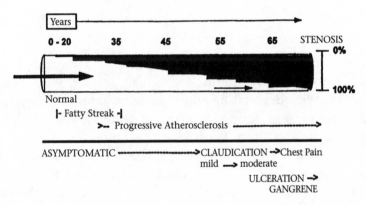

FIGURE 5

Over time, an artery's capacity for delivering blood can become compromised by the buildup of atherosclerotic plaque on its interior walls. Besides narrowing the channel through which blood can flow, plaque also hampers the ability of endothelial cells to produce nitric oxide from arginine, which is key to relaxing the encircling smooth muscle cells. From T.W. Rooke and A.T. Hirsh, "Peripheral Vascular Disease," in *Cardiovascular Medicine*, edited by J.T. Willerson and J.N. Cohn (New York: Churchill Livingstone, 1995). Reprinted with permission of W.B. Saunders Co.

Why should this be so? Begin with the fact that endothelial cells, like any other living tissues in your body, require a steady source of oxygen and nutrients. You might imagine they obtain this directly from the nutrient-rich and oxygenated blood coursing through the very artery whose inner diameter they border. If you lived on the banks of a giant river, wouldn't you be tempted to get your drinking water from the most obvious source?

In reality, endothelial cells ignore the mighty river in their front yard in favor of tiny backdoor rivulets. These so-called intimal vessels (called *vasa vasorum*) actually originate on the *outside* of the artery and weave through the vessel wall, penetrate through the surrounding smooth-muscle layers, then split into tiny creeks once they've reached the innermost layer where endothelial cells reside. This system works fine as long as nothing comes between the endothelial cells and the tiny arteriole "creeks" that supply them. Unfortunately, atherosclerotic plaque can do just this. Indeed, physiologists have discovered that even a thin "skim coating" of cholesterol-laden debris can block the access of endothelial cells to the blood supply they require to function.

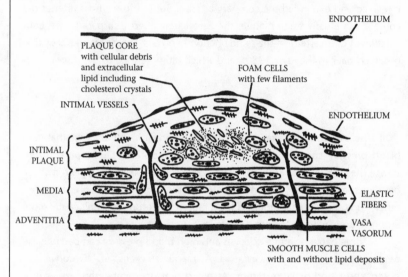

FIGURE 6
Atherosclerosis doesn't happen overnight. It usually takes decades to progress from initial fatty streaks laid down in early adulthood to the full-fledged, ragged, calcified plaques that can occlude arteries and serve as a magnet for clots. Studies suggest that arginine supplements can begin to reverse this process. From M.L. Buja, "Basic Mechanism of Atherosclerosis," in *Cardiovascular Medicine*, edited by J.T. Willerson and J.N. Cohn (New York: Churchill Livingstone, 1995). Reprinted with permission of W.B. Saunders Co.

As noted in earlier chapters, endothelial cells are absolutely critical to healthy vessel function because of their ability to make nitric oxide from arginine, which relaxes the surrounding smooth-muscle rings, in the process expanding both an artery's diameter and its blood-carrying capacity. When endothelial cells are blocked off from their blood supply, they can't make nitric oxide from arginine, the vessel constricts, and blood pressure begins to rise. Researchers have begun to show that even seemingly trivial amounts of plaque—like a wafer-thin dike— can result in such a barrier.

The medical journal *Circulation* recently featured an article that showed that the damage done to the endothelium by early-stage atherosclerosis can be roughly equal to the damage done to blood-vessel strips carelessly prepared for observation in a laboratory glass dish.[4]

Researchers injected the vessel-relaxing substance acetylcholine into the coronary bloodstreams of volunteer patients. In those who had no evidence of coronary atherosclerosis, the acetylcholine did what it was supposed to do, i.e., it relaxed and expanded the coronary arteries. But in those whose arteries did contain some early-stage plaque, the acetylcholine led to a paradoxical constriction of these arteries—the same phenomenon Drs. Furchgott and Zawadzki observed back in the early 1980s, and which ultimately led to the discovery of NO.

Death Spiral

If atherosclerosis can exacerbate high blood pressure, it's also true that high blood pressure can speed up the rate of atherosclerosis. One report, for instance, has shown that atherosclerosis is much more likely to appear in those parts of the circulatory system subjected to the highest blood pressure.[5] Another study showed that monkeys fed a high-fat diet formed significantly more arterial plaque when they also suffered hypertension.[6]

For some patients, atherosclerosis and high blood pressure can become like two snakes chasing each other's tail. As plaque thickens, ADNO conversion suffers and blood pressure climbs. As blood pressure climbs, the rate of new plaque protection escalates.

Fortunately, there is an effective way to interrupt this deadly spiral. Numerous studies now show that arginine supplementation can help ameliorate both problems, and in the process halt the synergy of these heinous co-conspirators. ADNO clearly lowers blood pressure, and it also clearly reduces cholesterol levels and prevents the LDL oxidation that is so critical to plaque formation.

Even better, an increasing cadre of researchers believe regular supplementation can do more than just prevent new damage—it can begin to reverse injury that has already occurred in blood vessels. In April 1997, *The American Journal of Hypertension* proclaimed as much in the clinical but nonetheless auspicious jargon of researchers: "Oral L-arginine had beneficial effects in hypertension . . . suggesting an improvement of endothelium dependent vasodilation."[7]

In laymen's language, the Arginine Solution means it's never too late to become young at heart.

80 mm Hg for diastolic pressure. You may be more surprised to learn that high readings, even astronomically high, are not necessarily harmful to health. Weight lifters, for instance, have had their systolic levels dramatically elevated in the middle of a power lift—with no ill effect on their health. Top aerobic athletes, such as elite marathoners, often see their systolic levels significantly elevated during a race, again without triggering health problems. If anything, the heart of a well-trained athlete becomes healthier than average due to a positive adaptation from his or her training workload. These adaptations reflect the heart's ability to remodel itself structurally, and in the process become a pump that's better suited to the jobs it's regularly called upon to perform.

In weight lifters, for example, the muscle walls of the heart chambers actually thicken slightly to withstand the high pressure demands. In elite aerobic athletes, the thickness of the heart walls remains unchanged, but the chamber size itself enlarges, allowing each heartbeat to propel more blood forward. Indeed, if you commit to a regular aerobic training regimen, your resting heart rate will probably decrease—evidence that your heart has become much more efficient and needs not beat as often to supply your body's needs. But go the other way—i.e., embrace the couch potato lifestyle—and even such a mild exercise challenge as walking up a short flight of stairs will likely cause your heart to race and blood pressure to soar and perhaps remain high after exertion is done.

There is a variety of other external factors that can cause blood pressure to spike. College students during exams and accountants during tax season have been shown to undergo stress-related increases in blood pressure. Even sexual arousal—hot-blooded passion and whatnot—can affect blood pressure. Clearly, it would be impossible, not to mention impossibly boring, to go through life without *ever* having elevated blood pressure at least some of the time. Our systems are designed for this.

Where people generally get into trouble health-wise is not with these acute, temporary rises precipitated by exertion or acute stress, but rather chronic elevation, where even at rest the pressure on your artery walls stays consistently high. In such cases, your heart itself has no choice but to make the best of a bad situation. To guarantee proper blood flow to your tissues, the heart must constantly work harder than normal, and over time this chronic, unrelieved workload can lead to an increase in its size. But unlike the adaptive thickening seen in some athletes, the enlarged hearts of longtime hypertensives become decidedly less healthy.

When the Heart Grows Too Big: LVH and Congestive Heart Failure

The powerful left chamber of the heart is particularly vulnerable to this pathological enlargement, a condition physicians call LVH (for left ventricular hypertrophy). Unfortunately, your blood pressure doesn't have to be tremendously high to begin triggering this change. A study published in the *Journal of the American College of Cardiology*, for example, looked at hypertensive employees at a variety of different work sites and found that 12 percent of those suffering only borderline high blood pressure already had LVH. In those whose hypertension fell in the mild-to-moderate category (see Table 3, page 57), the odds of having an enlarged heart climbed to one in five. For African Americans, the risk of developing LVH was higher than for whites at all levels of elevated blood pressure, but particularly at the borderline level. Perhaps most disturbingly of all, LVH— even in its late stages—tended not to present itself with telltale symptoms. Well over half of those whose heart had significantly swollen from hypertension had no idea whatsoever that such a change had taken place.[1]

You may be asking yourself, So what's the big deal about an enlarged heart? If your biceps gets bigger, it just means your arm has become that much stronger, right? Why doesn't the same thing apply to the heart? The problem with LVH is that it ends up interfering with, not strengthening, your heart's ability to pump blood. Indeed, if LVH becomes too severe and the heart too big, it ends up throwing off the precisely coordinated electrical communication between heart cells that allows them to contract in harmony. It's a little analogous to trying to keep up a hushed conversation with a friend who was once standing right next to you but has recently moved across the street. As you become more and more separated from each other, eventually even shouting won't let you hear each other anymore.

When the communication between heart cells really breaks down, it can cause everything from the abnormal beating patterns known as heart arrhythmias to a potentially catastrophic condition called fibrillation. The Latin root of this latter term means "bag of worms," and that's exactly what the fibers of a fibrillating heart look like: a wriggling, chaotic mess of uncoordinated heart muscles firing at random. You're probably familiar with the electric heart attack "paddles" long such a dramatic staple of TV shows from *ER* to *Baywatch*. These can sometimes shock the heart back to a normal rhythm, provided, that is, you survive long enough to get jolted.

Another physical change that occurs in a heart subjected too long to chronic high blood pressure is that it begins to require more oxygen to perform its workload, especially when this workload is high. This is particularly likely to occur in people with baseline blood pressure of 160/95 mm Hg or greater. Unfortunately, this extra requirement is often accompanied by a reduced ability of the coronary arteries to relax and deliver the additional blood flow. For patients like Stephanie M. undergoing abrupt stress at work or John R. trying to jog up a steep hill, the unmet demand for oxygen can trigger a heart attack and even sudden death.

All these changes to the heart can eventually so weaken its pumping ability that it no longer pumps sufficient blood to the body and the lungs. The diagnosis: congestive heart failure, a leading cause of disability and death.

Testing for Heart Disease

How can your doctor tell if you have heart disease? It's not always easy, because even the presence of multiple risk factors doesn't guarantee the condition, nor does the absence of these risk factors always assure heart health. Still, doctors need to start somewhere, and one good place is with your blood pressure. Indeed, a recent article in the British medical journal *The Lancet* found that elevated arterial blood pressure is one of the most important predictors for the risk of future heart attacks.

Using a stethoscope, doctors can get further clues about your heart's functioning by listening to the sounds it makes while beating. What sounds like an indistinct "thud-thud" to untrained laymen can actually reveal telltale blood-flow patterns to those who know what to listen for.

Patients diagnosed with hypertension or who are at risk for heart and blood vessel disease should also have a test called an electrocardiograph (ECG), which looks for abnormalities in the pattern of electrical activity arising from the heart. Though the ECG rarely diagnoses early-stage heart disease, it's pretty reliable in documenting more advanced cases. A more sophisticated and revealing form of ECG is a stress test performed while the patient is exercising or after his or her heart has been stimulated by injection to beat faster. Any impaired blood flow is picked up by monitors. If the stress test is equivocal, a radioactive scan (thalium or sestamibi) can be done in conjunction with the stress test to "light up" those parts of the heart that are over- or underfunctioning.

Another test, the ultrasound echocardiograph, uses the same basic technology employed by the sonar operators on submarines. But instead of looking for enemy subs via reflected sound waves, cardiologists use pulsed ultrasound waves to make out the movement and the structure of the heart itself.

Each year, new and ever more accurate techniques are coming on line to make the diagnosis of heart problems more specific and reliable. One widely used diagnostic tool, for instance, is the so-called stress-echo test, which combines an exercise stress test with an echocardiograph. Another new and extremely promising test is the "ultrafast CT-scan," which an early report from the American Heart Association called more powerful than the best available noninvasive test in predicting heart attack and other coronary disease episodes, even in apparently healthy people. The ultrafast CT-scan looks for the presence of calcium in plaque, an excellent indicator of late-stage atherosclerosis. Other high-tech approaches, such as MRI and PET scans, promise to help remove more of the guesswork from diagnosing heart disease. And when there is doubt as to the degree of atherosclerosis, the "gold standard" is still the invasive coronary arteriogram.

To be sure, which tests you may require to evaluate your heart is a decision best discussed with your doctor. Until then, focus your energies on healthy living and consider the benefits of the Arginine Solution. This will up the odds that no matter what test you may eventually undergo, it's going to reveal a healthy heart.

Undoing the Damage

Now for the good news. If you're suddenly wondering if you might one day be suffering a muscle-bound, oxygen-demanding heart whose cells cry out to one another—"What? Huh? I can't hear you! Come again?"—well, you can take heart. Researchers have demonstrated that aggressively treating high blood pressure via lifestyle modification and/or medications not only stems further ventricular enlargement, it can actually cause any LVH you now suffer to regress. You can, in other words, begin to reverse the damage.

Indeed, if taken long enough, all the standard antihypertensive drug treatments have been shown to have this beneficial heart-shrinking effect, and some, diuretics and beta-blockers included, can actually begin to undo the damage in a matter of weeks.[2]

The evidence is now also overwhelming that ADNO fosters similar changes, though it may require a somewhat longer time horizon to achieve results. Consider just one of the well-designed studies that is leading more and more clinical researchers to recommend the Arginine Solution to their patients suffering congestive heart failure and other consequences of long-standing hypertension.

In a 1996 paper published in the prestigious journal *Circulation*, researchers at the University of Minnesota Medical School investigated the use of oral arginine in the treatment of patients suffering heart failure. Their study, which was supported by a grant from the National Institutes of Health, cited earlier clinical trials that found that intravenous arginine significantly improved circulation in patients suffering advanced hardening of the arteries or recovering from heart transplants.

Specifically, the researchers wanted to determine if arginine administered orally as opposed to through injection could benefit their patients in three ways:

- Improve blood circulation at rest
- Increase the distance a patient could cover during a standard six-minute exercise walk
- Finally, improve a patient's overall quality of life

The patient volunteers were divided randomly into two groups. The first group received from 5.6 to 12.6 grams of oral arginine daily. The second group received a placebo. After six weeks, the groups were switched.

The investigators found that blood circulation, as measured in the forearm, markedly improved when a patient received the arginine supplement. Blood pressue also decreased, and the distance a patient could walk increased. Perhaps most encouraging of all, arginine significantly benefited a patient's score on the Living with Heart Failure Questionnaire, a standard measure of just how impaired, both physically and psychologically, heart patients perceive themselves to be. The change in scores indicated that these patients felt significantly better about their health while receiving arginine than they did while receiving placebos.[3]

What We Recommend

Thanks to studies such as this one, we're convinced that ADNO treatment will soon become more and more common in American health care. Because of its usefulness in checking hypertension, we believe supplemental arginine is an ideal *preventative* measure for presently healthy individuals at risk for heart disease who hope to safeguard their heart and prevent long-term pathological changes such as LVH and congestive heart failure. We also believe it can serve as an equally ideal *complementary* measure for those whose existing high blood pressure demands aggressive pharmaceutical treatment. For most individuals, a conservative but effective dose is somewhere from three to six grams per day, divided into three equal doses.

Alone or in combination with prescription medicines, this level of supplemental arginine will help to open your arteries, which will translate into a reduction in the chronic workload placed on your heart. This, in turn, will provide your heart with the rest it needs and deserves. It will therefore no longer need to make the best of a bad situation, but instead can revert to its healthier "pre-adapted" physiology. Instead of continuing to enlarge, your heart will actually start to shrink toward its normal size.

A note of caution: Be sure to ask your doctor if it is safe for you to take arginine supplements if you are also taking nitro-glycerin or nitrates in any form, or if you are using sildenafil, the anti-impotence medicine whose brand name is Viagra.

The bottom line: Examine the many lifestyle changes and nutritional modifications that can help improve your heart function, including a regimen of supplemental ADNO. If you take these steps and your heart is now healthy, it's much more likely to stay that way. And if your heart's been injured, you slash the risk of future heartbreak, even as you give yourself a chance to heal.

Chronic hypertension can lead to a dangerous form of heart disease distinct from the vessel-clogging form seen in athero-sclerotic cardiovascular disease. This so-called hypertensive heart disease has few if any warning signs, especially in its early stages. It hurts you by causing long-term changes to the physi-cal structure and functioning of your heart, which impairs its ability to pump effectively. These changes can include an en-largement of the powerful left ventricle, a degradation of the electrical communication between heart cells, which can lead to arrhythmias and fibrillation, and eventually congestive heart failure, or an inability to pump enough blood to where it is needed in your body.

Persistent high blood pressure is the first domino that sets all the others in motion. Regular use of supplemental arginine can help keep your arteries dilated and your blood pressure under control. In a person whose heart has not yet undergone detrimental changes, arginine can serve as an effective adjunct to preventative care. In a person whose heart has already been damaged by high blood pressure, arginine, sometimes bolstered by prescription medicines, can help stem further damage and in many cases help nudge the heart back toward its original, healthier anatomy.

10

Hitchhikers and Sticky Blood
How ADNO Clears Your Circulatory Highway

> Now as concerns the abundance and increase of this blood
> . . . those things which remain to be spoken of, yet when I
> shall mention them, they are so new and unheard of that
> not only I fear mischief which may arrive to me from the
> envy of some persons.
>
> —*William Harvey*

"As a competitive long-distance runner and an automotive engineer, I'm acutely aware of the need to supply my skeletal muscles with the fuel and oxygen that keeps them contracting at peak performance. I'm constantly reading articles in running magazines on everything from carbo-loading techniques to different training regimens designed to enhance endurance and VO_2 max. I'm doing, in other words, everything I can think of to keep my bodily 'machine' firing on all cylinders.

"I turned fifty last summer, and I know that my cardiovascular system has taken some hits. I smoked in my early twenties, an idiotic habit that, thank God, I was able to quit cold turkey after three years. My cholesterol used to be borderline high, too, that is, before I joined a masters' running club on my fortieth birthday. I believe my lifestyle over the past decade has begun to reverse the damage I once so carelessly inflicted upon myself. But I sometimes find myself wondering if there's any way I can give my body a further edge, not so much for health reasons per se, but just so I can run a 10K faster! It's like I'm driving a reasonably serviceable used Volkswagen now, but I sure would love to upgrade to a new Porsche.

"God knows I also wish my vascular system were as clean as a whistle and completely uncorroded by yesteryear's abuses. But I'm sure there's at least a little damage in there still. You can sometimes boost a car's performance with engine additives. I'd love to find an 'additive' to boost my own human engine."

—Charles M., 50

"One of the worst aspects of my heart disease is how easily I get winded just from walking. In fact, almost any exercise leaves me feeling breathless after only a couple of minutes. I used to wonder if there was something wrong with my lungs. My doctor says my lungs are fine—in fact, he tells me there have been aerobic athletes who competed successfully after *losing* a lung. She says I've got more than enough capacity to take in oxygen, it's my delivery system that's been injured. My heart and blood vessels, she explains, just can't supply enough blood fast enough to my muscles when they require extra oxygen and fuel. The result is I have to slow down, maybe even stop to rest in the middle of simple activities. A decade ago, I could climb mountains. Today, it's a challenge to climb a few stairs."

—Sheila J., 67

"After I suffered my first heart attack, my doctor recommended I start taking a baby aspirin every day. This would help thin my blood and prevent new blood clots from forming that could clog up my heart and lead to a second attack. After six months on the aspirin, I started to get stomach aches. I'm on so many different medications now that I couldn't tell which one of them, if any, was causing the pain, but I have heard that too much aspirin can sometimes cause ulcers in susceptible people. I'm going to be seeing my doctor next week, and hopefully he can give me something else to improve the situation. The problem I'm having with medicines, though, is that you can end up like that proverbial little old lady who swallowed the fly. You take something for one problem. It solves that, but causes another problem. So you take another drug to fix the second problem, and it causes a third one. They say that without chemicals, life itself would be impossible. I've got to tell you, when you're on a lot of chemicals, life gets pretty impossible, too."

—George S., 56

Who among us has not at times wished to possess more vigor, more stamina, more get-up-and-go? Certainly, the thought that we might somehow give our metabolic engines a tune-up is an appealing concept. In some regards, it's not even that far-fetched.

On the macro level, the body is truly a form of machine—infinitely more complex than the most expensive Ferrari, to be sure—but a machine nonetheless. It takes in fuel and oxygen, metabolizes these to create energy, then uses the resulting energy to power everything from movement and thought to immunity and reproduction.

Without sufficient nutrients and oxygen, the corporal machine quickly grinds to a halt like a car running out of gas. But even when the supply of these necessities is plentiful and access to them unencumbered, we can sometimes end up with less than optimal performance. For Charles, this can mean a disappointing time in a 10K road race. For Sheila, it can mean bone-deep exhaustion in the face of even a minor exercise challenge.

Why is this so? As Sheila's case so poignantly and dramatically portrays, it turns out that problems in the delivery of oxygen and nutrients can leave our cells with insufficient levels of these critical raw ingredients to create the required energy. This delivery system is, of course, our circulatory system. You may have in mind an image of blood laden with a cargo of oxygen and nutrients, all of it pumping along passively to your body's disparate tissues. Once it arrives at its designated destination, this cargo is jettisoned in exchange for metabolic wastes and by-products, which are then passively removed for discharging.

The reality is that there's absolutely nothing passive about the circulatory system's logistical role. An astonishing recent discovery about the part ADNO plays has convinced scientists that this process is, if anything, even more dynamic than they thought.

Breathe In

To understand better how this works, suck in a deep breath and hold it for a moment. The slight pressure you're now feeling against your rib cage is actually compressed air inflating tiny sacs deep inside your lungs. Each of these tiny sacs is, in turn, surrounded by capillaries containing red blood cells.

You've probably heard people say that blood "carries" oxygen. Inside each individual red blood cell—and we have an average of over 5,000,000 in every cubic millimeter of blood—there lurks a powerful "oxygen magnet" called hemoglobin. This complex protein allows us to pick up oxygen in the lungs and carry it to the cells that need it. Once the oxygen has reached its destination, the hemoglobin releases it and it becomes a magnet for carbon dioxide as well, which is then ferried back to the lungs for discharging. You can think of hemoglobin-containing red blood cells as miniature teamsters making an endless series of round trips, constantly switching back and forth between cargoes.

It sounds straightforward enough, and for decades, hematologists thought they pretty much understood the big picture of oxygen and CO_2 exchange. The thought that a previously undiscovered third gas might emerge to play a vital role in hemoglobin's functioning surely would have been dismissed as lunacy.

Until, that is, researchers discovered precisely this.

Serendipitous Discovery

In the early 1990s, researchers at Cornell University Medical College were searching for a way to use raw hemoglobin, as opposed to the hemoglobin packaged in red blood cells, as a

Blood's Busy Messenger

Scientists have discovered a major new function for the blood protein called hemoglobin. In addition to delivering oxygen (O_2) to the body's tissues and removing carbon dioxide (CO_2), it delivers a gas called nitric oxide (NO), which has important roles like regulating blood pressure.

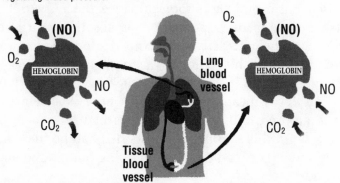

① In the lungs, hemoglobin that has already circulated through the body and has deposited its oxygen gives up the waste gases carbon dioxide and nitric oxide. Then it picks up a new load of oxygen and a differently bound form of nitric oxide **(NO)**.

② In blood vessels in tissue, the hemoglobin gives up its **(NO)** from one site and oxygen and picks up CO_2 and NO to take to the lungs to be exhaled.

Source: Duke University Medical Center

FIGURE 7

What controls blood flow? Copyright © 1996 by the New York Times Co. Reprinted with permission.

substitute for conventional blood transfusions. If they could get this to work, it would potentially solve a host of clinical problems, from avoiding the dreaded Rh blood-factor incompatibility in transfusions to precluding the spread of hard-to-detect infectious agents sometimes lurking unseen in whole blood.[1]

But when the investigators tried injecting the bloodstreams of laboratory animals with the raw hemoglobin, they witnessed an immediate and major problem. Instead of enhancing the blood's ability to carry oxygen, such injections resulted in a generalized constriction of an animal's arterial vessels, choking down blood flow. The effect was dramatic, and it left the scientists wondering what potent force could possibly be triggering such impaired circulation.

Subsequent experiments soon provided the answer. The injected hemoglobin, it turned out, was absorbing nitric oxide, i.e., the endothelium-derived relaxing factor we discussed in Chapter 5. Indeed, hemoglobin was doing such a great job of absorbing NO that it was actually sucking most of it out of circulation. This meant that relatively little NO remained to relax the arteries, and thus the arteries had no choice but to constrict. Until this finding, scientists had had no idea that the hemoglobin magnet could attract anything but oxygen and carbon dioxide.

The revelation was revolutionary enough that an article entitled "Surprise Discovery in Blood: Hemoglobin Has Bigger Role" made the front page of *The New York Times* on March 21, 1996.[2] In an age where designer molecules, from Prozac to Viagra, routinely adorn the cover of news magazines like so many chemical celebrities, hemoglobin's amazing "new" property showed that even an old-hat compound described for decades still has the capacity to astound. In a brilliant breakthrough paper published in *Science* in 1997, Dr. Jonathan S. Stamler and his colleagues at Duke University Medical Center went on to detail a wondrous three-way relationship between hemoglobin, oxygen, and nitric oxide that is now understood to be at the very heart of healthy circulatory functioning.[3] Dr. Stamler and his team showed that hemoglobin absorbs and releases nitric oxide depending on how much oxygen it is carrying.

The mechanism here is complicated. It begins in the lungs, where hemoglobin in the presence of NO is converted into a new molecule called S-nitrosohemoglobin, or SNO for short. SNO prevents nitric oxide from being readily expelled from the body, instead allowing it to hitchhike along with oxygen in the body's arterial highways.

Why ferry NO at all? It turns out that this biochemical hitchhiker can be released when needed to open up blood vessels. Say, for example, you're out jogging and the skeletal muscles in your legs have a dramatically increased need for oxygen. At rest, your femoral arteries and the smaller arterioles that branch off from them can easily meet your legs' oxygen requirements while remaining more or less undilated. But shortly after you hit the pavement, your leg muscles begin to cry out for more oxygen: Expand the pipes pronto—we're suffocating down here!

Ironically, when hemoglobin holds a lot of oxygen, it causes blood vessels to constrict. Two things, however, happen simultaneously to counter this and open vessels up. First, as the load of oxygen is reduced in tissues, the signal to constrict reduces. Second, and at the same time, SNO releases its NO hitchhiker, which snaps into action like a molecular traffic engineer, relaxing arterial smooth muscles. The result of this one-two punch: Vessels open and circulation increases. This ensures that the more oxygen a given tissue needs, the more it will get—courtesy of NO.

Which means your legs can keep on jogging without complaint.

As ingenious as this delivery system is, it can sometimes fail to work as designed. In earlier chapters we saw how vessel damage caused by atherosclerosis, smoking, high blood pressure, and other problems can impair the endothelial cell production of ADNO. We also showed how supplemental arginine can fortunately provide those healthy endothelial cells that remain with additional raw material to make more of the needed ADNO. Moreover, compelling evidence also suggests that arginine supplements can begin to heal those endothelial cells that have been damaged.

If atherosclerosis and other circulatory disorders only "bullied" endothelial cells, much of a patient's circulatory disorder would be on the road to resolution via the Arginine Solution. Unfortunately, these disorders can also trigger a second, altogether different problem for your circulatory system. Specifically, they cause a certain type of blood cell called a platelet to become "sticky." When this happens, these cells tend to clump together, forming clots that can impede blood circulation. In the worst-case scenario, you can end up suffering a catastrophic heart attack or stroke.

Fortunately, you don't have to just sit back and passively pray that the Grim Reaper passes you by. The same Arginine Solution that can help your endothelial cells function can also take a huge step toward reducing the dangers of sticky blood cells and clotting.

Of Platelets, ADNO, and Gridlock

A common misperception about the sole cause of heart attacks and certain kinds of strokes is that they occur when cholesterol-laden plaque, a sort of blood sludge, builds up so densely on the inner surface of a vessel that blood flow becomes totally "stenosed" or choked off, like an ancient water pipe that's finally become so corroded with mineral deposits that it will no longer drain.

This is not what always happens. Instead, a piece of the raggedy plaque buildup inside a vessel wall (thrombus) sometimes breaks off, spilling clotting debris into the bloodstream. This debris is known as an embolism, and once released into the blood, it can be propelled forward with each heartbeat. Eventually, it may wind up acting like a biochemical beaver dam. When the process involves a clot in a coronary or brain artery, it can starve these organs of the oxygen and nutrients they need to stay alive, resulting in a heart attack or stroke, respectively.

As is the case with so many aspects of our physiology, the tendency for blood to clot is most of the time a good thing—an adaptive response that we need to heal from injury. The next time you nick your finger, you can credit your innate ability to clot for keeping you from slowly bleeding to death. Indeed, until modern advances in medicine, hemophiliacs, who suffer from a genetic inability to form blood clots, usually died young from very minor injuries.

Ironically, it is this same healing mechanism gone awry that leads to nearly a million deaths from cardiovascular diseases each year in the United States. To understand how this happens—and how ADNO can help stop it—we'll need to focus for a moment on the body's smallest cells, i.e., your platelets, microscopic round or oval disks ("little plates") that lack a nucleus and circulate around in your blood for about ten days before dying. Whenever a blood vessel suffers an injury, from a cut finger to ruptured arterial plaque, platelets at the site of the injury clump together like tiny logs in a logjam. This effectively prevents blood from leaking out till the damage to the vessels can be repaired.

To be sure, if your platelets were perpetually clumping, your whole circulatory system would grind to a blood-crusty halt. Something has to trigger clumping when it's called for, while inhibiting it when there's no need. Nature, in its wisdom, has come up with an elegant mechanism for this, one that is no doubt familiar to anyone who's ever played with magnets.

Ordinarily, the exterior surface of blood platelets carries a negative electrical charge, which causes them to repel each other just as magnets of like polarity do. The inner surface of arterial blood vessels is also negatively charged, and as a consequence, platelets won't stick here either, unless, that is, something happens to alter the electrical charge.

It turns out that a number of blood-borne chemicals that are released when an injury occurs can alter that electrical charge, leading to a sort of "opposites attract" clumping. These chemicals include the histamine that makes you sneeze, the serotonin that affects your mood, and a complex molecule called PAF (for "platelet-aggregation factor"), which all work in complex ways to initiate and create blood clots.

Protecting the Heart by "Thinning" Blood

You've probably heard that so-called blood thinners are sometimes used to treat heart and hypertensive patients. This term conjures images of blood, thick as molasses, that requires diluting in some way so that it can course more freely through your blood vessels. In reality, this picture of blood thinners as a kind of physiological paint thinner is erroneous. What they really do is simply prevent platelets from becoming sticky and forming clots. A more accurate term for such medicine is anticoagulant.

Physicians and their patients have actually been benefiting from anticoagulant therapy since antiquity, though explanations for how this worked were often fanciful at best. For example, an ill patient would sometimes have his or her back covered with a species of bloodsucking leech (*Hirudo medicinalis*) that would quickly become engorged with blood. The good doctor would then pry off and discard the little feasters, confident they had sucked all the poisons from the patient's blood. The fact that the health of many of these patients sometimes improved seemed at the time to validate this toxin-removal theory. Indeed, so common was this practice that the word *leech* actually derives from the middle English term *leche*, meaning "physician."

Today, researchers have a better understanding of some of the mechanisms of "leech therapy." It turns out that leeches have an extremely potent natural anticoagulant called hirudin in their saliva. From the leeches' point of view, this is essential to their style of feeding because it prevents blood from clotting and thus keeps an uninterrupted stream of it flowing into their digestive tract. Natural hirudin as well as synthetic versions of it are now being studied in the fight against heart attacks. Squeamish patients take note: A hungry leech is no longer directly required to deliver the drug!

There's another potent anticoagulant that has been used since antiquity, though not necessarily because of its anticoagulant properties: the drug in the painkilling, anti-inflammatory compound aspirin. About ten years ago, physician volunteers were recruited to see if taking a single aspirin tablet containing 350 milligrams daily could affect the risk of heart disease and death by heart attacks. Researchers already knew that one of aspirin's many properties included the inhibition of platelet clumping. But was this inhibition simply an interesting lab finding, or was it actually powerful enough to affect cardiovascular health? The results of the physician study, which were published in 1997 in *The New England Journal of Medicine*, concluded that a daily aspirin does indeed have a significant impact on heart health, lowering the risk of heart disease and heart attacks.[4] Other researchers have also shown that aspirin can slash the risk of a second heart attack in patients who have already suffered a first heart attack. And because unchecked platelet clumping has also been implicated as one cause for chronic high blood pressure, aspirin and other anticoagulants may help in the treatment of hypertension as well.

Unfortunately, many of these anticoagulant drugs, aspirin included, can have pernicious side effects for many patients, side effects that can range from serious stomach bleeding to kidney damage. Indeed, further analysis of the same landmark physician study itself found that those doctors in a control group who received a placebo instead of aspirin had the same overall incidence of death as those who received the aspirin. How could this be, if the aspirin takers were enjoying such a comparative reduction of heart disease and heart attacks?[5]

Well, it turns out that the physicians on aspirin *increased* their odds of another, often fatal condition: hemorrhagic stroke, that is, unchecked bleeding into the brain. This kind of stroke is a prime example of where you need some protective blood clotting, but the anticoagulants have turned off the capacity to do so.

A more recent report from the Boston University School of Medicine cautioned that aspirin can irritate the stomach lining, causing sometimes severe upper gastrointestinal bleeding and, in rare instances, death.[6]

The bottom line: For some patients, "blood thinning" with daily aspirin can be a lifesaver, but for others it can result in a kind of disease substitution whereby reducing the odds of one bad outcome simply ups the odds of another.

If you are a blood donor, take heart! Regularly giving blood was found to be heart-protective, presumably because it reduces the volume of hemoglobin in the blood, a risk factor for heart attacks and stroke, according to the Framingham studies.[7]

ADNO: The Body's Safe and Natural Blood Thinner

The good news is that researchers have found another "blood thinning" approach that is equally effective in controlling platelet aggregation, but without the side effects of conventional anticoagulants from aspirin to leech saliva. This discovery came after Drs. M. W. Radomski, R. M. J. Palmer, and Salvador Moncada learned that platelets themselves contain their own form of the enzyme nitric oxide synthase, which lets them create NO from arginine.[8]

Why, they wondered, would platelets need to do this? Further research by these pioneers eventually suggested that the ability to form NO was a sort of "fail-safe" mechanism that limits the capacity of platelets to do inadvertent damage to the blood vessels they're designed to save. It's as if nature has equipped us with our own emergency clot-busters.

Alas, in people whose cardiovascular system is already severely damaged in multiple ways, the NO produced by platelets may sometimes be too little, too late.

But supplemental arginine can help a hypertensive patient's remaining undamaged endothelial cells produce additional NO to keep arteries open and prevent platelets from clumping and sticking to vessel walls. In fact, in 1994, researchers at the Hanover Medical School in Germany reported that intravenous arginine resulted in a 33 percent decrease in platelet aggregation—a very impressive result. Moreover, the researchers concluded that arginine inhibits platelet aggregation specifically "by enhancing nitric oxide formation."[9]

The effect of oral arginine on platelet "stickiness" is also surprisingly long-lived. In a report published in the *Journal of the American College of Cardiology*, cardiologists at Stanford University Medical School gave their patients with high serum cholesterol levels a daily dose of 8.4 grams of oral arginine.

After two weeks, these patients' platelets had become significantly less sticky. What's more, the beneficial effect remained undiminished for two more weeks *after* the supplements stopped. Indeed, it took a full eighteen weeks before the platelets returned to their pre-arginine levels of stickiness.[10] By the way, the patients experienced no significant side effects throughout the duration of the experiment.

If you are currently on a regimen of anticoagulant therapy prescribed by your doctor, you might want to consider discussing with him or her the possibility of adding three to six grams of daily arginine supplements to your treatment. If you haven't been prescribed blood thinners but have wondered lately if maybe taking a daily aspirin could be a prudent insurance policy for your future heart health, the same three to six grams of supplementary arginine could be a better, safer choice.

Not only will arginine help prevent your platelets from clotting, it will also provide your hemoglobin with more of the nitric oxide "hitchhiker" that is at the ready to hop off and dilate the blood vessels supplying tissues with a high demand for oxygen and nutrients. The Arginine Solution may just be the closest thing there is to an engine additive to rev up the performance of your human machine.

The delivery of oxygen from the lungs to body tissues, and the subsequent removal of carbon dioxide waste back to the lungs for exhalation is a complex event largely mediated by hemoglobin, an iron-containing protein found in red blood cells. Recent groundbreaking research has found that hemoglobin also binds to a third gas, nitric oxide. This is ferried along with oxygen and CO_2 and can be released when needed to dilate arterial vessels and thus allow more blood flow to tissues requiring extra oxygen.

Nitric oxide also figures prominently as a kind of fail-safe mechanism for blood platelets, the body's smallest cells. When a vessel sustains an injury, platelets become "sticky" and aggregate into clots that serve as miniature dams to stanch further blood loss. This protective mechanism can sometimes go awry in patients whose arteries have undergone narrowing and occlusion due to atherosclerotic plaque. Large blood clots can be deadly, especially when they occur in vital areas, such as the coronary arteries that supply the heart muscles or the arteries that feed the brain. Even a small clot can be dangerous, especially if it travels as an embolus and winds up clogging a small or narrowed artery. To prevent such an untoward outcome, heart patients are often prescribed anticoagulants to inhibit platelet stickiness.

Unfortunately, many of the conventional "blood thinners," including aspirin, can trigger other side effects, from stomach ulcers to hemorrhagic stroke (or bleeding into the brain).

Researchers have recently discovered that platelets contain their own form of an enzyme that allows them to manufacture nitric oxide when needed. This NO, in turn, can help open arteries and reduce the stickiness of platelets. Supplemental arginine holds great promise as a safe and natural anticoagulant, one that can help keep platelets in check when their "healing" function becomes overzealous enough to imperil cardiovascular health.

11

Just Say NO to Impotence
How ADNO Enhances Human Sexuality

Is it not strange that desire should so many years outlive
performance?

—*William Shakespeare*

"Do you know the difference between worry and panic? Worry
is the first time you can't do it a second time. Panic is the second time you can't do it the first time.

"My doctor told me this old joke a couple weeks ago when
I admitted to him I was having some problems performing in
the bedroom. I think his intention was to make light of impotence, to let me know it's not all that unusual a problem.
But when it happens to you, it's not that easy to see the humor
in it.

"On the plus side, medications can supposedly 'cure' almost
any erectile difficulty, even in guys who've suffered spinal cord
injuries. The new miracle drug Viagra has become more famous
than most movie stars. My doctor said he could write me a
prescription for a dozen pills if I want. Maybe I'll take him up
on it someday. At ten dollars a pill, Viagra is very expensive,
and my insurance probably won't cover it. It kind of rankles me
to think I need to 'pay for sex.'

"What rankles me even more is that I'm only fifty-two years
old, and it just doesn't seem right that I'd need to take drugs to

121

make love. I just wish there was something less drastic to bring me back to the way I used to be."

—Jerry F., 52

"I've been married for thirteen years, and I love my wife more now than ever. Our sex life has always been fulfilling, but lately I've had some difficulties maintaining an erection. The first time it happened was a couple months ago. After ten minutes of foreplay, I paused to put on a condom, and during this break in the action my erection faded. Try as I might, I couldn't get it back.

"My wife was very understanding, and she said that it was probably because I'd had a couple of beers earlier that evening. No big deal, she said. Things will work out fine the next time.

"Which they did, more or less. But I've got to say, it wasn't the most relaxing experience of my life. After 'failing' once, I felt all this tremendous pressure to 'pass' the next time. It was like sex had become this big final exam. Before, making love with my wife had always been this really great stress reliever for me. Now it had suddenly turned into this huge anxiety provoker.

"Some nights I find myself telling my wife I'm too stressed out from my job to feel very amorous. The truth is, I just don't feel up to 'taking the test.' She's really been nice to me, but I can tell she'd like things to be like they were before—natural, easy, relaxed.

"Sigmund Freud had his outdated theory about women and penis envy. Actually, in our marriage, *I'm* the one who's got the penis envy. And the penis I envy is the one I used to have."

—Hank E., 47

"I've read that menopause can cause women to suffer from vaginal dryness. I haven't gone through the change of life yet myself, and I don't expect to for at least five or ten more years. Still, I don't seem to be getting the same sexual response I did earlier in my thirties. Even when I'm really turned on by my husband, I sometimes can stay kind of unlubricated.

"We can usually overcome the problem with a water-based lubricating jelly. But it bothers me that I can't just respond naturally like I used to. I think it bothers my husband, too. Once he told me that he thought he must be a really boring lover. He tried to make a joke out of it, but it broke my heart to think he was blaming himself for my inability to respond.

"With all the publicity surrounding Viagra, it's now just accepted that a man's impotence is most often a physical problem. I wish we could all become a little more enlightened about things that affect women. You may not hear the word *frigidity* much anymore, but I don't think the concept's gone away. It's like a man's sexual problems have all been destigmatized as a medical problem, but a woman's sexual issues still seem linked in people's minds to a cold, screwed-up, prudish psychology. I'm not any of these things!

"Sometimes I wonder if I'm suffering from the same physiological problem that causes a man to become impotent. I've read that women during arousal experience increased blood flow to the genitals the same as guys. I do have high cholesterol. Maybe this is part of the problem. I find myself hoping they'll start making a Viagra for women."

—Elsa W., 38

In 1985, a fifty-three-year-old man made love to his wife, and in the process gave her a terrible headache. The episode would eventually prove quite enlightening to scientists studying the complex biology of erectile function.

To understand why, consider the fellow's medical history. At the age of thirty-eight, he'd been diagnosed with severe coronary atherosclerosis. His physician recommended he undergo bypass surgery as a preemptive measure against an almost certain heart attack. The man agreed. But despite successful surgery, two and a half years later he suffered a heart attack anyway. He survived, but it left him with recurrent chest pain due to permanently impaired coronary blood flow.

At this point, his doctor prescribed twelve-hour-release transdermal patches containing nitrates—sort of a high-tech variation on an age-old traditional heart-pain remedy of placing a nitroglycerin tablet under the tongue. When worn on his chest, the patches slowly and steadily leached chemicals through his skin to dilate coronary blood vessels, allowing more blood to flow to his heart muscle, and thus better managing the pain of his angina pectoris.

Unfortunately, these same patches that took away heart pain also gave him bad headaches, a well-documented and common side effect of this treatment. On his own, the man decided to experiment with the placement of the patches, moving them from his chest to his legs. This seemed to eliminate his headache, but he wasn't sure exactly why. Was it just because the patches were now more distant from his head? Or could it be that the skin on his legs was thicker, so less of the nitrates was entering his bloodstream?

To find out, the amateur scientist decided to place the patches on an area of his anatomy that was at once reasonably far removed from his cranium but definitely not thick-skinned. The result of rubbing the nitrate patch on his penis was as dramatic as it was unexpected. Within five minutes, he had become erect. Sex with his wife quickly followed. Several minutes after this, *she* reported developing one of the worst headaches of her life.

The man later confessed his homemade experiment to her. Though her headache had by then abated, she was less than impressed by his armchair science, and, in fact, strongly discouraged any more investigation in this area. He later related the episode to his doctors, who were intrigued enough to publish the odd episode as a case study in a medical journal.[1]

Their article was titled, straightforwardly enough, "Transdermal Nitrate, Penile Erection, and Spousal Headache." The doctors knew well that nitrate caused increased coronary artery blood flow and that nitrate, in this instance, must have seeped into the underlying vasculature of the penis, increasing blood flow there, too. Evidently, the wife had gone on to absorb some of her husband's nitrate, which then triggered her headache by dilating blood vessels in her head. Because the arginine/nitric oxide mechanism had not yet been discovered, however, the doctors back then were much more interested in the particulars of the wife's headache than the oddities of the man's erection.

They summarized their findings in the *Annals of Internal Medicine* this way: "This case illustrates two previously undescribed points concerning topical nitrates: their ability to induce vasodilation and resulting erection. . . . The authors personally doubt that further research in this area will be done." Since it was not known yet that any topical compound could induce erection, and certainly no one suspected that nitrate could possibly do this, this conclusion is somehow akin to telling the Wright brothers that all they managed to do was imitate birds.

In hindsight, of course, the man's erection would prove to be highly significant, a truly revolutionary discovery despite the fact that it initially got lost in the shuffle. Indeed, the idea that an externally applied chemical substance could affect erectile function prefigured the sea change to come in the conventional understanding of erectile function.

Most practitioners at the time still embraced the notion that impotence was largely a psychological, not a physical, disorder. Indeed, famed sex researchers William Masters and Virginia Johnson had declared in their influential book, *Human Sexual Inadequacy*, that 90 percent of all impotence is caused by some form of psychological or emotional conflict.[2]

There had been, of course, a few other lines of evidence emerging in the early 1980s that cast doubt on this "all in your head" notion of erectile dysfunction. In 1982, for instance, researchers had first developed the penile-brachial index, which compares blood pressure in the penis to blood pressure in the arm. Impotent men had a large disparity between the two measurements; healthy men did not. This form of diagnostic testing led to a new appreciation of the role of circulation in healthy erections.[3]

This was further bolstered by accumulating epidemiological data that showed much higher rates of impotence in men who smoked and/or suffered from diabetes, atherosclerosis, high blood pressure, depression, or took common prescription drugs that affected circulatory function.

One of the most eye-opening attempts to prove that vasodilation was key to erections occurred at the infamous 1983 American Urological Association meeting. While presenting a paper on this topic, British neurophysiologist Dr. Giles Brindley pulled down his pants midlecture, injected himself in the penis with a long-acting alpha-blocking drug, and paraded around the room with an erection, proving the paradox that erection requires blood-vessel relaxation.

Nevertheless, it would be years before a new appreciation for the role of blood circulation in erectile functioning came into mainstream accceptance. And it would get its final shove thanks to a 1992 discovery by urologists at the University of California in Los Angeles.

It's a Gas

When a man becomes sexually aroused, you might imagine that the muscles in his penis are working overtime. Actually, precisely the opposite is true. As counterintuitive as it may seem, erections can only occur when the smooth muscles in the penis *relax*. As long as these muscles remain constricted, the penis paradoxically stays flaccid. The reason for this becomes clear when you realize that erections are not the result of muscular flexing but rather of blood engorgement. The more blood that is able to flow into the penis and expand it, the firmer the erection will be.

The gatekeepers for such blood flow, it turns out, are smooth muscles in the spongy tissues of the penis. When these are constricted, they keep the arterial inflow of blood squeezed down to a trickle, much like squeezing a garden hose. But when these same smooth muscles are triggered into relaxing, it's akin to opening the hose back up. Blood from the penile arteries rushes in, quickly filling two expandable reservoirs inside the penis called corpus cavernosa.

To be sure, an erection would be short-lived if something didn't also effectively prevent this blood from draining back out as quickly as it entered. As the corpus cavernosa swell like two parallel water balloons, they press against penile veins that normally drain blood out. The more blood-swollen the cavernosa become, the greater the pressure on the veins, which now slows the rate of outflow. The result is an erection that's both rigid enough and long-lasting enough to allow for intercourse.

Though the general hydraulic physiology of erections had long been well understood, scientists were not at all certain what complex biochemistry was orchestrating this precise balance of vascular inflow and outflow. As Dr. Giles Brindley had dramatically demonstrated a decade earlier, a shot of vasodilating drugs could trigger blood engorgement. But what innate chemical did the body itself use to give itself such a shot?

In the early 1990s, urologist Dr. Jacob Rajfer and other researchers at UCLA discovered that in the healthy penis, blood inflow is triggered when nerve endings release the short-lived gas nitric oxide.[4] This is the same NO that had so recently emerged as the chief natural relaxant for the smooth-muscle rings in arteries themselves. The researchers determined that NO, like a tipped domino, initiates a series of biochemical reactions in the penis that ultimately engorge it with blood and allow it to remain erect.

In declaring NO the 1992 Molecule of the Year, the editors of *Science* referred to the pivotal discoveries at UCLA when they wrote: "This year scientists proved definitively that in men, NO translates sexual excitement into potency by causing erections. The pelvic nerves get a message from the brain and make nitric oxide in response. NO dilates the blood vessels throughout the crucial areas of the penis, blood rushes in, and the penis rises to the occasion."[5]

But if NO action causes healthy erections, could NO problems be at the root of impotence? In a report in *The New England Journal of Medicine*, Dr. Rajfer and colleagues suggested the answer was a resounding yes. Defects in the NO system, they suggested, could prevent sufficient inflow of blood or, alternatively, could cause blood to leak out prematurely, in either case quashing an erection. Dr. Rajfer suggested that up to 80 percent of impotence in American men was directly attributable to some form of NO failure.

What could cause these "defects" in the system? At the time, the investigators thought the likeliest culprit was a failure of the enzyme that produces NO in the penis. It was possible, they suggested, that this deteriorates with aging, which would explain the fact that age itself is the single greatest risk factor for impotence. No one at the time suggested that because the body makes its nitric oxide supply from L-arginine, it might just be possible to remedy low penile NO production by boosting the available arginine supply.

Dr. Arthur L. Burnett of the Johns Hopkins Hospital in Baltimore hinted at such a possibility in *The Journal of Urology* when he wrote, "Nitric oxide is synthesized as a byproduct of the catalytic conversion of L-arginine . . . by the enzyme nitric oxide synthase (NOS). . . . Nitric oxide exerts a significant role in the physiology of the penis, operating chiefly as the principal mediator of erectile function. Alterations in the biology of nitric oxide likely account for various forms of erectile dysfunction."[6]

Other investigators soon began exploring the potential of supplemental L-arginine as a treatment for impotence. One of the first of such studies appeared in 1994 in *The International Journal of Impotence Research*. Here, researchers reported the results of a clinical trial in which fifteen impotent men were given a very modest 2.8 grams of oral L-arginine daily for two weeks; fifteen other impotent men were given identical-looking placebo capsules.

Keep in mind that the average American consumes 5.4 grams of arginine daily from such foods as meat, poultry and fish, dairy products, eggs, and cereal. Thus the "treatment dose" was really modest, barely a 50 percent increase over normal intake. Despite this, six of the men receiving L-arginine showed significant improvement in erectile functioning. None of the men on placebos improved.[7]

Since then, other publications in medical journals have re-

Of Sleep and Female Potency

O ne of the most interesting aspects of human sexuality hasn't emerged from Masters and Johnson–style laboratories where human test volunteers have sex while simultaneously rigged up to a battery of sensors that measure everything from pelvic-floor muscle twitches to skin moisture levels. Rather, it's come from the nation's sleep labs, which for years have shown a nightly "rise and fall" cycle of erection followed by flaccidity in sleeping men. Indeed, healthy guys experience up to a half dozen discreet erections each night, mainly during periods of dream sleep. Some of these nocturnal erections can last up to an hour or longer.

This phenomenon has been so well documented that it's led to a simple home test to determine if a man's impotence is primarily physiological or psychological. Before going to sleep, a patient is instructed to encircle his flaccid penis with a ring of connected postage stamps, gluing the overlapping ends together with the adhesive already on the stamps. In the morning, if this ring is still intact, it means he didn't have any nocturnal erections, and the problem requires a further diagnostic workup by a urologist. If the ring has been broken, it means he is at least physically capable of having an erection during sleep.

More recently, sleep researchers have discovered that it's not just men who undergo nightly changes in their sex-organ blood-flow patterns. Sleeping women undergo nearly identical changes as well. To be sure, blood engorgement of the vaginal tissues may be harder to see than the changes in a penis as it becomes erect, but more and more doctors now believe that a healthy sexual response in women is as dependent on a well-functioning vasculature as it is in men. Vaginal lubrication, for instance, is just one example of a process that's highly dependent on ample blood flow in the urogenital arteries.

No one knows for sure why the sex organs undergo so much activity while we sleep. When awakened during a period of arousal, some volunteers report having erotic dreams, but more often the process doesn't seem linked to them. One theory is that it's a way of ensuring that plenty of oxygenated blood and nutrients will make their way to sexual tissues.

Given the fact that men and women have the same basic "sexual hydraulics," researchers are now actively investigating the use of drugs, like Viagra, as a way of enhancing female sexuality. Though more research remains to be done, it is possible that women could achieve the same benefits as men via the Arginine Solution. Taken regularly, arginine supplements promise to enhance blood-flow patterns to the female sex organs, restoring what might one day soon be commonly known as female potency. Hopefully, more research into this overly neglected area will soon be forthcoming.

confirmed that this effect is real. Arginine supplements seem to boost erections in the full spectrum of men, from the completely healthy to those suffering from advanced circulatory disease.

In men without erectile problems, for example, arginine seems to strengthen and prolong erections. In those with occasional failure, it can reduce the frequency of such occurrences. In men with more serious so-called vascular impotence due to advanced atherosclerosis, hypertension, or diabetes, dietary arginine can gradually begin to reverse damage and rejuvenate penile function.

This is, of course, not an overnight cure by any means. Given the time it takes to build up significant vessel damage, it seems unlikely that anything could reverse it overnight. But if arginine is taken regularly and consistently, key changes to blood vessels and the endothelium will occur. Dr. Anoop Chauhan of Cambridge, England, was quoted as saying in the *Medical Tribune* (Internist and Cardiologist Edition) in December 1995: "We have demonstrated for the first time that you can reverse this [aging] effect with L-arginine."

The Invention of a Best-Seller

Pharmaceutical firms determined to come up with revolutionary new impotence cures are likely to give a wide berth to L-arginine despite its considerable track record. The reason: Arginine is a nonpatentable food supplement. Drug companies face considerable costs in researching and testing new medications in order to secure FDA approval to market them. With-

Recipes for Impotence

Researchers today know that upwards of 80 percent of impotence cases can be linked to purely physical problems, from cardiovascular and neurological ailments to smoking and drug abuse. In a landmark study that surveyed the sexual functioning of more than 1,000 men, many of these factors were precisely quantified.[11] Some of the key statistical findings from this and other studies show that:

- Age was the single greatest factor in becoming impotent. Two-thirds of forty-year-olds reported no problems with impotence; only one-third of seventy-year-olds could make that same claim. Despite this correlation, age per se does not cause impotence; healthy men can maintain potency into their nineties and beyond. Rather, the chronic diseases that frequently accompany old age tend to be the real cause of impotence.
- So strong is the link between early impotence and atherosclerotic heart disease that some cardiologists have already begun considering impotence before sixty as an early biomedical marker for future heart problems.
- Smoking dramatically increases the risk of impotence. In one study, one-third of the men smoked, and almost two-thirds of these had experienced erectile failure. In men with heart disease, smoking ups the odds of impotence by fully three times compared to heart disease patients who don't smoke. A report in the *Journal of the American College of Cardiology* suggests that smoking is so ruinous to sexual health because it damages the endothelial cells, which are the key to blood flow in the penis. The good news: Supplemental arginine appears able to reverse this in many men.[12]
- Diabetes afflicts over 15 percent of adult men in the U.S. population. From one-half to two-thirds of these men will eventually be diagnosed with organic impotence. Evidence continues to accumulate that diabetes impairs sexual function, in part, by depressing nitric oxide levels. Once again, supplemental arginine may be able to reverse some of the damage.
- In some studies, dangerously high cholesterol can be a prescription for impotence. Of the 5 percent of men with the highest cholesterol, fully one-third are impotent. Other studies find that an even more important factor than high total cholesterol is low levels of so-called good HDL cholesterol. Men aged forty to fifty-five who participated in the Massachu-

setts Male Aging Study saw their odds of being impotent escalate from 6.7 percent to 25 percent as HDL dropped from 90 to 30 mg./dl.

- High blood pressure is also a strong risk factor for impotence. Indeed, 15 percent of men diagnosed with hypertension are completely impotent. Once again, the likely mechanism at work is an impairment of nitric oxide production, which can be corrected by supplemental arginine.
- Nearly 90 percent of men who ranked highest on measures for depression reported moderate to severe impotence.
- Contrary to conventional wisdom, low testosterone levels are an exceedingly rare cause for impotence. Even though testosterone levels do tend to fall with advancing age, the vast majority of elderly men continue to have more than enough to maintain normal sexual activity. When problems do occur, it's almost never because of testosterone deficiency. What's more, even if you do take testosterone supplements, it's unlikely to improve your ability to perform—just your desire to do so. When it comes to sexuality, testosterone affects libido, not penile circulation and erection.
- Finally, a wide range of prescription and "recreational" drugs, from beta-blockers to beer, can affect erectile performance. If you develop erectile difficulties and are on a medication, check with your doctor or pharmacist to see if drug chemistry could be contributing to the problem.

out the light of patent protection at the end of the development tunnel, it just doesn't make economic sense to underwrite such costs.

Fortunately for stockholders in Pfizer, Inc., the drug company that brought the blockbuster drug Viagra (sildenafil citrate) to market, ADNO is only one step in a serpentine biochemical chain reaction that creates and sustains erections. To be sure, ADNO alone can improve erectile function in many men. But just because it works effectively doesn't mean a drug company can profit dramatically from its sale.

Corporate profits require proprietary formulations, a compound that a company can legitimately claim to have invented, thus justifying a decade or more of noncompetition through patent protection. In their quest to find such a proprietary drug,

Pfizer researchers cleverly focused their efforts on another part of the "ADNO to blood flow" biochemical pathway.

By analogy, you can think of such a pathway as an amazingly complicated variation on the old song that informs us that "the ankle bone's connected to the shin bone, the shin bone's connected to the knee bone," and so forth.

Here is a quick and simplified overview of the erectile process:

Step 1. Sexual stimulation causes a variety of nerves originating in the brain to start firing.

Step 2. Once stimulated, these nerves cause the release of the neurotransmitter acetylcholine in the penis.

Step 3. This acetylcholine, in turn, causes the endothelial cells in penile arteries to begin producing NO from L-arginine, a transformation that occurs thanks to the enzyme nitric oxide synthase.

Step 4. Once created, NO triggers the release of another naturally occurring chemical called "cyclic guanosine monophosphate." Cyclic GMP, it turns out, is one of many potent vasodilating chemicals found in the human body.

Step 5. As cGMP levels build, the smooth muscles of the penile arteries relax, the vessels dilate, and increased blood flow causes swelling of the corpus cavernosa, producing an erection.

Step 6. Even as NO continues to build up cyclic GMP, another enzyme begins to break it down. This enzyme, phosphodiesterase, appears to act as a brake on the overall system, preventing erections from becoming excessive or permanent. Though this might sound like a fantasy to some lust-addled fellows, such a state—which physicians call priapism—can lead to permanent damage to erectile tissues.

Step 7. Following climax or other cessation of the sexual stimulation, the penile nerves stop firing and the nerve end-

An Eccentric Neurotransmitter

S imply put, a neurotransmitter is a form of chemical switch that turns things on or off. It is typically released by a nerve cell in the tiny gap that separates it from a neighboring nerve or muscle fiber.

Acetylcholine, which starts the sequence of penile erection, is an example of an off-switch neurotransmitter because it signals smooth muscles to turn off their contraction and relax, letting blood flow into the spongy tissue of the penis. After acetylcholine has done its job, a specific enzyme called acetylcholine esterase breaks it down into its component "building blocks" and stores these in a special nerve storage vesicle. Later, if more acetylcholine is required, the building blocks can be reassembled and released again.

Researchers have discovered dozens of different neurotransmitters, and virtually all of these have their own unique form of breakdown enzyme and storage vesicle. One major exception to this pattern is nitric oxide, which scientists have only recently learned can act as a neurotransmitter in addition to its many other roles in the body. For many researchers, this was initially hard to believe because NO lacks a storage vesicle and an enzyme to break it down.

Evidently, it doesn't need one. NO breaks down into nitrates on its own after only a few seconds, the chemical analog of an old general who simply "fades away" when his job is done. When more NO is needed, the body simply manufactures more, provided there's a sufficient arginine supply.

ings cease releasing acetylcholine. Without the acetylcholine signal, the endothelial cells cut back on NO production. And without the NO signal, no more cGMP is produced. What little cGMP remains free-floating is soon broken down by phosphodiesterase. The result: the smooth muscles of the penis blood vessels once again contract, and the penis goes into its nonaroused, compact state.

Given this convoluted flow-chart arrangement, it's easy to see how erections might potentially be affected at a number of different stages. Remember the man with heart disease who rubbed his nitrate patch on his penis, got aroused, and gave his wife a horrible headache? Nitrates, like arginine, are an excellent source for making NO. It now appears the man was boosting his erection by simply enhancing the above Step 3. His wife absorbed some of these nitrates vaginally, which led to her headache. How much happier they both might have been if he had used a condom—or better still, simply ingested arginine, which can help produce erections without causing headaches in either party.

The fact that topically applied nitrates did prove stimulating, however, was not lost on researchers questing for an impotence cure. In the late 1980s, for instance, investigators at Queens University, Kingston, Ontario, reported giving thirty impotent men a tube of ointment each. Half received a nitroglycerin ointment, and half received a placebo. Each man was then shown an X-rated videotape. Men whose ointment contained nitroglycerin enjoyed a 50 percent increase in the diameter of the penis.[8] Those on placebo did not benefit.

Numerous subsequent trials have reported similar successes with a host of nitric oxide donors applied to the penis via a patch or ointment. In explaining the success of such products, the *British Medical Journal* reported that such agents "are absorbed topically and generate nitric oxide either spontaneously or after metabolism in smooth muscle. Nitric oxide . . . [causes] local relaxation of corporeal smooth muscle. This results in increased filling of the corpus cavernosum with blood and consequently impairment of venous outflow, thereby causing penile erection."

Such approaches even appear helpful to men with long-standing, chronic impotence. Indeed, a hospital study in Denmark provided nitroglycerin patches to men who averaged sixty years old and had each been impotent for at least five years. All patients found they were able to achieve erections with the help of the patches. The main drawback was headaches, though these tended to diminish with continuous use.[9]

Going back for a moment to our "Seven Steps to Erection" biochemical pathway, it's easy to see how other impotence "cures" work by targeting different stages in the process. One drug currently under study, for example, is a sublingual tablet that works directly on the brain, in effect amplifying nerve signals to the penis. Other drugs, such as papaverine, prostaglandin E1, and VIP, are potent vasodilators that can be injected directly into the spongy tissues of the penis or inserted through the urethra. They produce erections by directly relaxing blood vessels.

Viagra works by an entirely different mechanism. Pfizer researchers created a drug that blocks the enzyme phosphodiesterase. Without this enzyme to put the brakes on cyclic GMP, levels of this potent vasodilator can build unchecked. For impotent men whose ability to create NO has been impaired by damage to the endothelium, what little NO they can produce slowly but steadily triggers cGMP.

Undoubtedly, future drugs will continue to come on line that will allow impotent men to trigger erections by a variety of novel techniques. No doubt these, like their current-day predecessors, will be expensive and subject users to the potential for peculiar side effects. Case in point is a decidedly bizarre symptom seen in some men taking relatively high-dose Viagra: They suffer blue-green color confusion. It turns out that the phosphodiesterase Viagra so successfully blocks in the penis also plays a role in color perception. For reasons that aren't yet fully understood, certain susceptible men taking Viagra can have trouble telling blue from green. This effect appears to go away once Viagra treatment stops, but it's too early to know if long-term problems might be associated with its use.

The Natural Solution

Human physiology is not unlike a bewilderingly complex and interconnected ecological system. "Cures" for one problem can sometimes have far-reaching consequences for seemingly unrelated systems, much as the use of DDT to kill crop-damaging insects came close also to driving the American eagle to extinction. It is for this reason that doctors dating back to Hippocrates strive first and above all else "to do no harm."

Part of this approach means taking only enough medicine needed to treat a given problem. Many Americans subscribe to the faulty, dangerous belief that "if a little bit of medicine helps you, a lot of it will help even more." Another frequent misperception is that a newer or more expensive drug is always better.

Nutritional therapy, from the vitamin E in nuts to the isoflavones in soy protein, occupies a somewhat uncertain position in the public consciousness. On the one hand, most of us know full well the benefits of eating a healthful diet—and the drawbacks of living on junk food. But when we actually become sick and develop frightening symptoms, from angina to impotence, it's all too easy to relegate nutrition to the back seat. Give us *real* drugs with *real* effects, we demand. Health food's fine when you're healthy, but now's the time for real medicine.

But the nutritional supplement arginine *is* real medicine. The *Harvard Health Letter* reported that the amount of nitric oxide produced in the penis, and thus the ability to have an erection, is directly related to the availability of L-arginine.[10] If you're currently suffering from some measure of erectile dysfunction, or if you just want to keep things operating properly in the future, we strongly urge you to give oral arginine supplements a try first. As researchers across the globe have affirmed in leading journals, arginine is not some mild placebo with only marginal effects on penile blood flow. Rather, it has been shown time and again to provide your body with the one critical item it most requires to function optimally: nitric oxide.

To be sure, in some cases, renewed erections may be restored within minutes of a penile injection of powerful vasodilators. Oral arginine, on the other hand, may take up to an hour— comparable to the time it takes for Viagra to enter your system. But taken regularly over several weeks, three to six grams of daily arginine offers substantially more than the "quick fix" of these well-publicized and heralded drugs. It can slowly but steadily begin to rejuvenate penile arteries, provide your stressed endothelial cells with more of the precursor they require to make NO, and generally give your whole cardiovascular system a tune-up.

Think of the Arginine Solution as a "chronic tonic" for your entire cardiovascular system, which includes your penile plumbing, too. If, after a fair trial, you find arginine hasn't restored potency to the extent you hoped it would, you can always try pharmaceutical drugs at that point. But studies have shown that you may never need them.

Erections during sexual arousal are the result of a complex biochemical chain reaction. A key step in the process occurs when endothelial cells in penile blood vessels increase production of nitric oxide from arginine. This, in turn, ends up triggering blood flow into the cavernous chambers of the penis. As the pressure builds, it presses against penile veins, reducing outflow and resulting in an erection.

As recently as the 1970s and 1980s, impotence was thought to be principally a psychological problem. The medical community now recognizes that the majority of cases are caused by physical disorders that contribute to a failure of the arginine/nitric oxide mechanism in the blood vessels of the penis. While numerous kinds of nitric oxide donors have been successfully used to promote erection instantly, oral supplementation of arginine may, in most cases, work just as well, though it may take somewhat longer to achieve results.

We recommend that men—and women alike—go one step farther. Don't just use arginine as a prelude to sex. If you are at risk for, or if you suffer from, problems with impotency, consider taking three to six grams of arginine *daily* for long-term benefits to your sexual functioning.

Arginine supplements are available from a number of distributors. The supplements may also be found under various brand names, such as Real Health Laboratories' VasoRect Clinical Strength Formula, in most stores where health products are sold. See the appendix for a list of some of these distributors.

12

A Call to Arms
ADNO and the Immune System

They say that the first inclination which an animal has is to protect itself.

—Diogenes Laertius, circa 200 A.D.

"It seems like I am constantly catching colds or picking up little stomach infections that last a couple of days before running their course. I haven't always been so prone to getting sick, but my new job is super stressful, and my boss is the kind who flies off the handle ten times a day and takes it out on everyone around him. I started doing aerobics for an hour every day after work, and it's a great stress reliever. I also do some weight lifting and running. But sometimes I feel this exercise runs me down a little, too. There are weeks when it seems I've painted a giant bull's-eye on my back—an open invitation to every cold virus, flu bug, and food-poisoning bacteria to just come on over and get me."

—Liza G., 40

"I've been teaching elementary school for eleven years, and you'd think my immune system by now would have seen every kind of virus known to man. A lot of my fellow teachers tell me that early in their careers, they got sick a lot, too, catching all the stuff going around at school. But after a few years, they

139

seemed to develop some resistance. I haven't. In the winter, especially, I get sick practically every other week. Nothing serious, thank God, but it's a drag to be constantly fighting off something. I keep hoping they'll come up with a cure for the common cold, but until that day, I wish there was something that can give me an edge in the battle against the bugs."

—Larry V., 34

"I've spent much of the past year training for the Boston Marathon, which it has been my dream to run since I was a teenager. Between now and race day, I want to make sure I put in enough miles to get in top shape, but not overtrain to the point of exhausting myself. I'm averaging between forty and fifty miles a week. I've also been really watching what I eat—lots of complex carbohydrates, not too much meat or fat. I feel like I'm doing all the right things. But I took the same steps two years ago, as well, and what did it get me? Three days before that year's race, I caught a bad strain of flu. By race day, my temperature was a hundred and three. I almost ran anyway, but my wife threatened to have me committed. There's an old expression that goes, Once stung, twice shy. The truth is, I'm really scared I could get sick again this year. It was probably just a random event that won't repeat itself. But it sure would be good if you could train more than just your muscles and cardiovascular system. Wouldn't it be great if you could get your immune system in top shape, too?"

—Mike K., 47

The human immune system has long inspired military analogies, and for good reason. From constant skirmishes with hundreds of known cold viruses to periodic all-out wars waged against life-threatening infections, our immune-system cells are in a constant state of preparedness against hostile forces that would do us harm.

On the enemy's side, there's a seemingly endless onslaught of microbial malefactors intent on colonizing us and prospering at our expense: bacteria, viruses, fungi, parasites. Add to this rogues' gallery the traitors from within—some of our own cells grown wild, proliferating out of control, somehow turned cancerous and deadly.

On our side, we rely on an incredibly sophisticated and adaptive defense system that, when stimulated into counterattack, moves with a logistical grace that makes Desert Storm seem like child's play. Our immune forces have numerous specialized soldiers. We have cells that scout out and identify enemy invaders, quickly sounding the bugle call to rally an initial response. We have natural killer (NK) cells that hunt down and destroy the enemy. We have a variety of phagocytes—literally, "cell-eaters"—including the macrophages that gobble up, dissolve, and spit out the rubble of our vanquished foes.

We also have specialized "suppressor" cells, sort of like biochemical MPs, whose sole purpose is to keep their fellow soldiers from going berserk and attacking *us*. We even have special "intelligence officer" lymphocytes that learn to recognize each specific adversary by the protein uniforms they wear—and create tailor-made antibodies to neutralize them in the future.

As further evidence for the complexity of our immunity, consider this: Researchers have to date described five specific antibody subtypes—one to recognize and remain ever vigilant

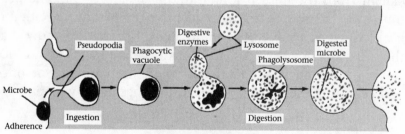

Phases of phagocytosis.

FIGURE 8

Specialized immune cells called macrophages can gobble up microbial invaders, digest them, and eliminate them as threats to the body. From Gerald Tortora and Nicholas Anagnostakos, *Principles of Anatomy and Physiology*, 4th edition. Copyright © 1983 by Biological Sciences Textbooks Inc., A&P Text, and Ella Sparta, Inc. Reprinted by permission of Addison Wesley Educational Publishers.

toward the most common infections; one to stand guard in the body's mucous membranes, from the nose and throat to the vagina and rectum; one to fight germs that cause blood cells to clump; one to stimulate the others into producing more antibodies; and, finally, one that mediates allergic reactions.

Now add in the confounding fact that not all foreign microbes in the human body are harmful. Quite the opposite, in fact—we host numerous beneficial bacteria, allies we need to stay healthy. Some of these, for instance, help us digest our food. Others synthesize essential vitamins. If we are to thrive, our immune system must somehow be able to distinguish the good "bugs" such as acidophilus from the bad, attacking the latter without mercy while simultaneously sparing the former. For the most part, it executes its manifold responsibilities with astonishing efficiency.

But the above simplistic description, of course, only begins to hint at how comprehensive and complicated the immune system is. From IgM antibodies to "helper" T-cells, understanding all the nuances of interrelated activity is challenging even for those investigators who have devoted their lives to studying this.

Fortunately, you don't need a doctorate in immunology to benefit from the unseen forces lurking inside us all. The next time you get a fever—a usually adaptive temperature rise that is itself triggered by special immunological proteins—know that there is actually a "heated battle" taking place inside you. Once you've recovered, you can thank your immune cells for once again fighting the good fight—and for once again winning.

Arming Immune Warriors

In the wake of the AIDS epidemic, the study of human immunology has received unprecedented scientific scrutiny. One quirky observation that had long puzzled microbiologists was that humans and animals alike routinely pass out significantly more nitrates in urine than they take in from dietary sources. By the 1980s, investigators were starting to suspect that the immune system itself must somehow be involved in this process.

This suspicion was fueled by several different findings. In an experiment using mice, injections of bacterial debris into the bloodstream quickly provoked a dramatic rise in urine nitrate levels. Moreover, physicians saw a similar increase in people who had suffered an infection, a severe injury, or were victims of acute blood poisoning.

It was during this same time period that researchers, working on separate but parallel tracks, were first discovering the role of nitric oxide in the relaxation of blood vessels. They observed that the more nitric oxide produced for this reason, the more the body expired NO from the lungs. Could the immune system, as well, somehow be manufacturing nitric oxide?

In 1985, Drs. D. J. Stuehr and M. A. Marletta published a landmark paper in the *Proceedings of the National Academy of Sciences* that for the first time provided direct proof that macrophages—one type of the immune system's "cell-eaters"—had their own form of the NO enzyme that lets them manufacture nitric oxide from arginine.[1] But the big question remained: Why?

In the coming years, more and more evidence mounted that NO might serve as something of an immune system "bullet" capable of killing off microbial invaders and cancerous cells alike. In 1991, for instance, cancer surgeons in Scotland published a study in *The Lancet* that showed that thirty grams of oral arginine given to cancer patients in divided doses for three days stimulated a 91 percent increase in the ability of their lymphocyte natural killer (NK) cells to neutralize target cells.[2] Moreover, research into the body's inflammatory response suggested that macrophage-manufactured NO plays other vital roles as well.

Tissues on Fire

You've almost certainly experienced inflammation firsthand on your skin following a cut or scrape. Depending on severity, inflamed tissues become red, swollen, noticeably warm to the touch, and often extremely tender. In some cases, the combination of swelling and pain can leave a body part temporarily unable to function, an experience familiar to anyone who's suffered a badly sprained ankle.

Painful as it can be, inflammation is actually one of the ways your body attempts to repair damage and destroy any opportunistic infections that may have used the injury as an opportunity to invade. The inflammatory process progresses in predictable stages, which, in somewhat simplified overview, look something like this:

Immediately following the injury, nearby blood vessels dilate, allowing more blood to flow to the affected area. Along with this dilation, the permeability of vessel walls also increases. This allows certain components in the blood, which are ordinarily too large to pass through the vessel walls, to cross over into adjoining tissues. Small immune-system cells, for instance, can now slip through to reach the site of injury.

Both these effects—increased blood flow and increased vessel wall permeability—are triggered by chemical signalers, including ADNO produced by macrophages as well as histamine, serotonin, and other substances that are released by injured and dying cells. Thanks to the greater permeability, fluid continues to seep into the injured tissues faster than it flows out, and this leads to a form of swelling that doctors call edema.

As the inflammatory response intensifies, platelets arrive on the scene along with more immune-system cells and a clot-forming substance called fibrinogen. In response to different chemical signals, the shape of each platelet changes, and they begin to clump together, forming a kind of makeshift dam around the injury. As fibrinogen seeps through the vessel walls into the injury proper, it converts into an insoluble substance called fibrin. Between the platelet clumping and the fibrin, the infection is effectively sealed off. Then enzymes begin to dissolve dead tissues for removal by the lymph "drainpipes." This limits any spreading of microbes while also stopping the internal bleeding. In cases of massive trauma so severe that the body can't stop this interior blood exodus fast enough, patients can die of internal hemorrhaging.

Though a myriad different chemical reactions take place during every pitched battle, scientists have learned that ADNO plays several especially critical roles in a healthy immune reponse. As indicated earlier, ADNO released by macrophages stimulates increased blood flow and vessel wall permeability that shunts front-line immune troops to the battlefield—this facilitates the mop-up and elimination of dead cells, toxic by-products, and other debris when the conflict resolves.

The antioxidant properties of ADNO, which were discussed in detail in Chapter 8, help inactivate the surplus of free radicals that form at an injury site. ADNO also triggers the release of prostaglandins, hormonelike chemicals that intensify blood clotting and further stoke the inflammatory process. These prostaglandins, in turn, lower our pain threshold. We might not like it much at the time, but a healthy dose of pain is actually a great way to make sure we take it easy for a while, and prevent further injury till the wound has healed.

Shooting to Kill

One of ADNO's most intriguing roles, however, is its ability to serve as a kind of immune-system bullet (see Figure 1, page 19). Researchers now believe that small bursts of ADNO fired by macrophages combat our microscopic opponents in at least two separate ways. In some cases, nitric oxide gas interferes with iron-containing molecules crucial to cellular respiration. This kills the enemy by poisoning it. Among the common infections that nitric oxide is known to kill by this mechanism are:[3,4]

- *Salmonella,* a bacteria that causes countless cases of food poisoning each year. Victims suffer sharp abdominal cramps and severe diarrhea.

- *E. coli* 0157, the infamous bacterial killer responsible for the deaths of several children who ate contaminated and undercooked hamburgers.
- *Helicobacter pylori,* the same bacteria discovered by two Australian doctors to cause most cases of peptic ulcer, and which has recently been implicated in migraines and heart disease.
- *Chlamydia,* a widespread, sexually transmitted bacteria that can cause symptoms ranging from urethritis to sterility.
- *Candida albicans,* a common form of yeast infection.

Besides this direct poison-gas attack on germs, ADNO provides a second mechanism to neutralize infectious invaders and possibly tumor cells as well: its ability to interfere with the enzymes necessary for DNA replication in harmful organisms. By throwing a monkey wrench into this process, ADNO can keep infectious agents and cancer cells from reproducing, which puts a major dent in their ability to hurt us. Let's look at this process further.

Traitorous Tissues

Cancer, of course, is not a single disease but rather a host of specific diseases that have in common the uncontrolled proliferation of different body cells. So-called benign cancers are usually not fatal, partly because they tend to stay put in their original location. Malignant cancers, on the other hand, tend to break off and spread throughout the body via the bloodstream or lymphatic system, in effect seeding new colonies far from the original "primary" tumor. Interestingly, most cancer deaths occur not because of the original cancer but rather from its prodigal offspring that have taken root at secondary sites.

Theories abound for what triggers cancer. Some researchers believe that cancer cells are quite common and that they pop up spontaneously in virtually everyone. Our immune systems, thank God, usually destroy them quickly, stemming the tide.

Another theory holds that in antiquity, different viruses invaded and fused with the DNA of our distant ancestors, forming so-called oncogenes (literally, cancer genes) that have been passed on via genetic inheritance to the modern day. A highly publicized example is the so-called breast-cancer gene, the presence of which significantly increases the odds of developing the disease. Oncogenes, it should be pointed out, don't doom their owners to cancer. Rather, some researchers believe they need the right mix and intensity of carcinogens, from cigarettes to ultraviolet radiation, in order to "wake up" and trigger uncontrolled cell growth.

Other researchers point to modern-day viruses, which have clearly been implicated in certain specific forms of cancer. Kaposi's sarcoma, for example, is the most common kind of cancer seen in HIV-infected patients. In 1994, investigators used a high-tech DNA-gene sequencing process to show that a previously unknown human herpes virus was the root cause of this cancer. Since then, this same virus, designated HHV-8 because it was the eighth human herpes virus to be identified, has been linked to other cancers, including multiple myeloma, which affects plasma cells.

Yet another theory holds that our cells are slated to die after so many reproductions, a process called programmed cell death. This is thought to be regulated by structures called telomeres that adorn the ends of our chromosomes and, in a sense, keep them intact the way the plastic ends on shoelaces keep these from unraveling. In normal cells, telomeres shorten with every reproduction, and once they're gone, the cell dies. But in cells that have become cancerous, this shortening doesn't occur. That's why some researchers believe cancer-cell reproduction can theoretically go on forever.

Immortality, at least on the cellular level, seems to be a synonym for cancer.

The Legacy of Helen Lane

Basic American cancer research has made use of this immortality since 1951, when a patient named Helen Lane died after a long bout with cervical cancer.[5] Her doctors at Johns Hopkins Hospital in Baltimore removed cancer cells from her cervix and cultured them in a glass dish filled with nutrients. This cell line, named HeLa after her, has continued to survive and replicate ever since in research laboratories the world over. Forty-five years after Helen Lane's death, her cancer cells show no sign of giving up the ghost.

Helen's legacy has provided researchers with an invaluable opportunity for studying the cancer-killing potential of different drugs. Trials of promising agents tend to take place sequentially. First, investigators try out a formulation on cancer cells in vitro, literally "in glass"—like the HeLa cell line. If it proves effective here, researchers next test it in vivo—i.e., "in life"—by giving it to laboratory animals with induced cancer. Again, if the drug continues to show promise—without also triggering unacceptable side effects—the researchers determine dosage levels that are likely to be safe and effective in humans. The final step is a graded series of clinical trials to see first if the drug is indeed safe, and second if it does offer any significant benefit to human patients.

Research on ADNO's effect on cancer has followed this step-by-step process. Long before researchers had any inkling that macrophages can make NO bullets capable of disabling tumor cells, scientists had already observed that an ample supply of L-arginine was essential to a robust immune response to cancer cells. After first demonstrating this in vitro, scientists in 1975 reported in the highly regarded journal *Cancer Research* that dietary arginine supplements seemed to boost cancer-fighting immune cells in rats. In their study, they fed 120 rats a standard diet enriched with arginine.[6] They fed 90 other rats the same diet but without the arginine supplements. They then injected all the rats with a known carcinogen. By the time the rats were sixteen weeks old, about 25 percent of those receiving arginine had developed cancer, averaging one tumor per subject. Most of these tumors were a benign form known as fibroadenoma.

The control group did not fare nearly so well. Nearly 90 percent had developed cancer, averaging five tumors apiece. Even worse, the majority of these tumors were a highly malignant variety known as adenocarcinoma.

A spate of follow-up research at various laboratories demonstrated several general principles. An arginine-rich diet inhibits tumor growth in animals, *but it does not completely prevent tumors from arising after exposure to a carcinogen.* Furthermore, when dietary supplements cease, the protective effect also ends, suggesting that continuous supplementation is required to keep tumors under control.

As much as we'd like to think that science marches forward in a logical, step-by-step fashion, in reality it's a much messier business, full of serendipitous findings, false hopes, and dead ends. Another element in the ADNO and cancer story had actually taken place well over a century earlier in 1882, when doctors first began noticing a very odd finding.[7] Their cancer patients who also suffered from bacterial infections seemed to have enhanced resistance to their cancer. This, like the relationship between arginine and tumor growth in lab rats, was another of the many puzzle pieces that had not yet been assembled into a cohesive picture.

Flash forward to 1987, when scientists at the Kaplan New York University Medical Center and the Suntory Biomedical Research Institute in Japan jointly announced the discovery of a substance released by immune cells that combats tumors.[8] They called this substance tumor necrosis factor, or TNF. Though it failed to serve as the long-sought cure-all for cancer, TNF nevertheless proved to be an invaluable part of the body's cancer-fighting forces. In 1988, an international team from the United States and France demonstrated that NO stimulates the production of TNF by lymphocytes and macrophages.[9]

By the early 1990s, researchers at the University of Utah had shown that arginine was the only amino acid that macrophages in mice need to inhibit the reproduction of certain cancer cells.[10] Cornell University scientists subsequently revealed the specific mechanism at work: The macrophages were using arginine to manufacture NO, which they then "shot" at tumor cells. Once inside the tumor cell, NO disabled a key enzyme necessary for the reproduction of cancerous cells.[11]

In the years to follow, numerous studies have examined the effect of ADNO on a spectrum of different cancers in vitro and in vivo, but much more work needs to be done to determine its role in the clinical treatment of cancer patients. In many cancers, arginine seems to hold considerable promise as an adjunct to traditional care because of its ability to arm immune cells with NO bullets.

One important caveat should be considered. It's been known since the 1970s that supplemental arginine can stimulate the release of human growth hormone, or HGH, a fact that weight lifters have long hoped provides an edge in building muscle bulk. Another conceivable benefit of HGH is that it may even help to retard the aging process. We'll be looking at arginine and HGH more closely in the next chapter. For now, you should note that some researchers believe that a surplus of HGH can fuel the growth of certain cancers. See Chapter 14 for more on this and other caveats.

Healing Wounds by Boosting Arginine

One area of clinical practice where the Arginine Solution is playing an increasingly important role is wound healing.[12] From helping patients overcome trauma more quickly to expediting recovery after surgery, many doctors have begun administering ADNO to patients to boost the body's innate restorative powers.

Wounds invariably pose a risk of infection and inflammation. Slice open your skin in the tropics and you're more susceptible to infection, which could lead to sepsis. But even in an astringent hospital setting where doctors compulsively scrub down with antimicrobial soaps and use sterilized instruments to incise patients inside a sterile environment, wily bacteria and other microbes can still sometimes gain a foothold inside us.

Once a wound does become infected, the immune system fights back as best it can. A regimen of antibiotics can aid in this fight, but more and more microbes are proving resistant to the best drugs pharmaceutical science can throw at them. If antibiotics don't always work, how can we up the odds that our immune system will vanquish our adversaries?

Scientists studying wounds have long observed that the affected tissues often have uncommonly low levels of arginine in them. Dr. Adrian Barbul, using rat subjects as a model for human injury, provided them with extra arginine and found that this significantly reduced inflammation and speeded up the rate of healing.[13] In later work, Dr. Barbul showed that such enhanced recovery took place regardless of whether the L-arginine was given by injection or orally. He concluded that arginine supplementation was not just a case of replacing a vital nutrient, but rather it worked by providing injured tissues with a substance that specifically contributed to the healing response.

Spurred by these reports, doctors at the University of Pennsylvania School of Medicine decided to give arginine a trial in patients undergoing surgery and at a high risk for postoperative complications. In the days leading up to surgery, as well as for seven days afterward, one group of patients received 25 grams of oral L-arginine daily. A second group received a similar dose of the amino acid glycine instead of L-arginine.

Compared with the glycine group, the arginine group showed evidence of significantly increased immune-cell activation that began before the surgery, and by day seven following the operation, it had climbed to fully three times that seen in the glycine patients.[14] Other studies soon followed, including one published in *Critical Care Medicine* that demonstrated shorter hospital stays and reduced infections in critical-care patients who were provided with supplemental arginine. According to an article in the *Journal of Surgical Research*, dietary supplementation of L-arginine stimulates immune-system response and may prevent immune-system failure in injury and in trauma victims.[15]

It now seems clear from animal and human studies alike that the Arginine Solution boosts immunity by providing macrophages and other immune cells with the raw material needed to make ADNO. As effective as this appears to be in helping us overcome infections once we've developed one, it seems equally promising that regular arginine supplements can also keep our immunity well armed and fine-tuned during healthy times as well. Though the case is not yet definitively proven, evidence mounts that the Arginine Solution taken regularly can help nip small infections in the bud, preventing small flare-ups from turning into a full-scale war.

The human immune system is an inordinately complex defensive army of specialized cells and chemical weaponry that, when operating properly, protects us from a wide array of infectious agents and cancerous cells alike. From antibodies to tumor necrosis factor, different immune soldiers use a host of specialized chemical bullets to recognize and neutralize the vast ranks of our microscopic enemies.

In the mid-1980s, researchers first learned that the body's lymphocytes and macrophages—or "cell-eaters"—have a special form of an enzyme that allows them to make nitric oxide from arginine. Later researchers showed that macrophages can use NO to poison the internal metabolism of enemy cells, or to interfere with the ability of these adversaries to reproduce their DNA. NO is now known to be an effective killer of a wide variety of common infectious disease agents, from *Salmonella* to *Chlamydia*. NO bullets fired by macrophages and other immune cells also have the power to zap some tumors. And clinical studies have shown that oral and infused arginine can help wounds heal more quickly.

Because of its ability to arm the immune system with a key kind of bullet it needs, the Arginine Solution holds great promise for keeping our defensive forces in top shape—and, by extension, us as well.

13

A Cornucopia of Complementary Cures
ADNO's Effect on Other Major Maladies

> For full indeed is earth of woes, and full the sea; and in the
> day as well as night diseases unbidden haunt mankind,
> silently bearing ills to men.
>
> —*Hesiod*

Throughout this book, we've tried to inform you about the
many ways the Arginine Solution can serve as a tonic for your
body's most critical physiological systems. From tuning up your
heart and cardiovasculature to providing your immune system
with the necessary firepower to combat infections, ADNO is
fast emerging as one of mankind's most beneficial "nutraceutical" agents.

To be sure, if you can keep your major body systems operating optimally, that alone will go a long way toward preventing
many of the secondary "spin-off" diseases that afflict so many
people today. Take, for example, nephritis—aka kidney disease—the eighth leading cause of death in people sixty-five or
older. Though a small percentage of cases are caused by faulty
genetics, exposure to toxins, or even too much grueling exercise
performed while dehydrated, the vast majority of cases result
from damage inflicted on the kidneys by years of chronic high
blood pressure, atherosclerosis, and/or diabetes.

If you currently suffer from kidney disease, ADNO may or
may not directly impact your kidney cells—we just don't know

yet. But ADNO undoubtedly will help to treat many of the harmful underlying disorders, like high blood pressure, that have for so long put a burden on your body's crucial blood-filtering organs. Perhaps even more promising is the possibility that ADNO can help prevent kidney disease long before it has a chance to develop. If your kidneys are *not* now diseased, a regimen of daily arginine supplements begun today may well help inoculate you against future problems.

In the rest of this chapter, we will be examining some of the many other disorders for which the Arginine Solution is currently under active investigation as a treatment. For some of these, ADNO's benefits are once removed; i.e., it helps fix the primary problems that give rise to secondary problems. In other cases, ADNO works more directly on the disease process in question. Either way, its potential as both a therapeutic and a preventative agent now seems very promising indeed for a wide array of health problems. As Dr. Jonathan S. Stamler of Duke University so succinctly summed it up earlier, "Nitric oxide does everything, everywhere. You cannot name a major cellular response or physiological effect in which [ADNO] is not implicated today."[1]

Diabetes: The "Passer Through" with Honey

Diabetes mellitus is the seventh leading cause of death in the United States, killing nearly 57,000 people every year. Victims of different forms of diabetes share an inability to keep their blood-sugar levels from rising to dangerous levels. Such elevation, in turn, can lead to progressive damage to the heart, large blood vessels, capillaries, kidneys, nervous system, and brain.

Diabetes also promotes atherosclerosis and can trigger life-threatening seizures by lowering a patient's blood pH balance toward acid. Poor circulation in the extremities predisposes many diabetic men to impotence. In men and women alike, diabetes can result in gangrene in the hands and feet, a catastrophic infection that can require amputation of the affected limb. Diabetics can even become blind due to damage to blood vessels in the eyes.

This devastating disease derives its name from two Greek words: *diabetes,* meaning "passer through," and *mellitus,* meaning "honey." The conjoined name is apt. Indeed, when blood-sugar levels become sufficiently high, the urine of a diabetic becomes sweet. Our hats are off to whoever first discovered this.

The two most common forms of diabetes are Type I, or insulin-dependent diabetes, which usually develops in children and young adults; and Type II, or non-insulin-dependent diabetes, which afflicts primarily obese adults over the age of forty. Type I occurs when a person's pancreas is unable to secrete sufficient insulin, a substance that regulates glucose in the blood and urine. Type I diabetics must self-administer insulin by injections for life. In Type II diabetes, often called adult-onset diabetes, the pancreas is usually working fine, but the body itself becomes "resistant" to insulin, so that greater than normal amounts are necessary to maintain normal blood-glucose levels.

How ADNO Can Help Diabetics

When serum sugar levels climb high and stay that way too long, it sets off a number of harmful biochemical reactions in the blood. Excess sugar, for instance, can bind to hemoglobin, a damaging process known as glycosylation. Glucose can also react with certain proteins in the blood, producing megamolecules that can destroy fragile capillaries and reduce a diabetic's life span by as much as one-third.

One tissue that appears particularly hard hit is the endothelium that lines arterial blood vessels. Researchers at Harvard Medical School have found that blood flow in the forearms of diabetics is significantly lower than that seen in nondiabetics. Such poor circulation appears to be due, in large part, to impaired nitric oxide produced by damaged endothelial cells.[2] The good news: As we saw in Chapter 7, supplemental arginine clearly seems capable of restoring at least some of the arterial system's capacity to circulate blood.

For reasons that are not entirely understood, diabetes also greatly accelerates hardening of the arteries in many patients. One likely contributor to this is "lipid peroxidation"—that is, when blood fats such as LCD are turned "rancid" by oxygen free radicals. As discussed earlier, as cholesterol-laden plaque builds, so does blood pressure, which further exacerbates diabetic complications. In a sense, hypertension, atherosclerosis, and diabetes are like evil triplets in a pernicious "mutual admiration society." Each separate disorder complements the others in a vicious spiral of bodily vandalism. ADNO can interrupt the spiral at many points, not the least of which is its ability to reduce lipid peroxidation. In one study, thirty patients with diabetes mellitus received two grams of oral L-arginine a day while a diabetic control group received placebos. After three months, the arginine group showed signs of significantly decreased lipid peroxidation compared to the controls—a major benefit in the fight against atherosclerosis.[3]

In the heart muscle itself, long-standing diabetes frequently triggers an abnormal accumulation of collagen fibers, which are akin to scar tissue. Cardiologists know that local injury to the heart, as well as an excess of oxygen free radicals and platelet clumping, can cause these same changes in the hearts of nondiabetic patients. Supplemental arginine in such patients appears to help reverse some of the collagen deposition—might the same hold true for diabetics as well? Early work, though not definitive, indicates the answer may well be yes.

In 1994, researchers at the University of Vienna demonstrated that oral arginine supplements significantly reduced collagen accumulation in the heart muscle of diabetic mice. This benefit occurred at dosage levels roughly comparable to those used in treatment of human heart patients—around 7.5 grams a day in a man weighing 150 pounds. After another series of animal studies, Dr. Ian I. Joffe and his colleagues from Beth Israel Deaconess Medical Center in Boston concluded that cardiac dysfunction in diabetes mellitus is due to impaired availability of nitric oxide.[4]

Arginine may have an even more direct benefit, especially for those suffering the adult-onset form of the disease. Researchers have long known that different amino acids stimulate our various glands into releasing hormones. In highly promising work done at Northwestern University Medical School, the amino acid arginine was shown specifically to increase levels of the hormone insulin in Type II diabetics, most likely via a direct formation of nitric oxide in the pancreas. Not all researchers are yet convinced that nitric oxide in pancreatic cells stimulates insulin production, and clearly much more work remains to be done to determine arginine's role in an overall treatment plan for diabetes.[5]

But for now, the future looks bright. Researchers at the Medical College of Wisconsin have demonstrated three facts that reinforce the validity of the Arginine Solution as a complement to conventional care. First, blood levels of arginine are reduced by diabetes. Second, oral supplements can bring these levels back up to normal. And third, this boosts nitric oxide production, which restores blood vessel function and improves other pathological changes caused by diabetes.[6]

ADNO and the Brain

Put your fingertips together then spread your hands apart. The space created will give you a pretty good estimate of the size of your brain. Weighing in at under three pounds and sporting the consistency of firm oatmeal, this miracle of complexity is made up of billions of nerve and support cells that together affect the functioning of virtually every system in your body, from sexual performance to immune response.

The healthy brain consumes 25 percent of the body's oxygen supply and an astonishing 70 percent of its blood glucose. It also produces a bewildering array of chemicals. Cut off blood supply for more than a few minutes, and brain cells quickly begin to die. Even if blood flow is just slightly reduced, the resulting reduction in oxygen, if chronic, can contribute to a spectrum of mental disorders, from impaired thinking to disorders of senility.

Just as ADNO plays a key role in relaxing coronary arteries to guarantee a plentiful blood supply to your heart, so does this mechanism now appear to regulate blood flow to your brain. A 1993 animal study in *Brain Research* showed that inhibiting the enzyme used to make NO from L-arginine caused constriction of the arteries supplying the brain. The body responded by elevating blood pressure to make sure enough blood still made it through. When the researchers then infused their animal subjects with arginine, the vessels dilated and blood pressure normalized.[7]

But what about blood flow within the brain's famously convoluted gray matter? You've probably seen high-tech brain scans that show different regions of the brain "lighting up" depending upon what kinds of activities a person is asked to perform. What these colorful images are actually revealing are changes in regional metabolic activity that accompany different cognitive tasks. The areas that are working hardest, in other words, are also using up more oxygen and glucose to do their jobs. Those areas that are "on break" require a reduced supply.

Brain researchers have for years been intrigued by the brain's ability to form these small functional activity networks and to shunt blood preferentially, via arterioles and capillaries, to the precise area where it's most required. In the vernacular of students of the cerebrum, this phenomenon is known as "cerebral microcirculation during neural activity." So what exactly regulates it?

To find out, neuroscientists applied low-intensity nerve stimulation to the paws of rats. As expected, this quickly produced increased metabolic activity in a specific area of the rat's brain. It also produced a 30 to 40 percent dilation in the arterioles that supplied this area. Remarkably, no such dilation occurred in adjacent arterioles that branched off from the same major artery and fed brain cells only a small distance away. The author of the study, Dr. C. Iadecola, concluded that the agent of such precise vascular control was none other than nitric oxide being produced by activated brain cells.[8]

But ADNO has other functions in the brain, too, besides orchestrating blood flow. The way different nerve cells "communicate" with one another is through the release of specific messenger chemicals called neurotransmitters. These are typically secreted in the synapse—the tiny gap that separates the end of one nerve cell from the beginning of a neighbor. Serotonin, noradrenaline, and dopamine are just three of the more famous examples of neurotransmitters, levels of which can be affected by drugs ranging from antidepressants like Prozac to Parkinson's treatments like levodopa. Recently, neuroscientists have learned that nitric oxide functions as a neurotransmitter, facilitating communication among nerve cells whether they are connected via synapses or not (see Figure 1, page 19).

No one can yet say for certain what roles the ADNO neurotransmitter plays. One possibility may be the activation of memory storage. When you file a memory in long-term storage—say, your first kiss—the brain undergoes a complex process called long-term potentiation, or LTP. In a sense, it's not unlike writing yourself a note, then tracing it over backwards to make sure the letters are nice and dark. This reverse tracing, neuroscientists suspect, requires a "retrograde messenger"—one that can somehow work backwards to reinforce and "darken" nerve connections originally laid down when your lips first met. According to researchers at Stanford University School of Medicine, NO may well be this retrograde messenger. In fact, they were able to show that inhibiting the enzyme that makes ADNO in the brain interferes with long-term memory storage.[9]

Other brain researchers have begun to examine the role of ADNO in diseases such as Alzheimer's and Parkinson's. In patients suffering either of these disorders, there is frequently a significant reduction in the nitric oxide being produced in their brain. Recent articles in both *Nature* and the *Journal of Neurological Sciences* offered evidence that this reduction may hamper memory storage and reduces blood flow to the brain.[10,11] The latter may at once contribute to and be exacerbated by deposits of a specific kind of plaque, called beta-amyloid, that is a hallmark of several degenerative brain diseases including Alzheimer's. This plaque, though chemically different from the atherosclerotic plaque that clogs heart arteries, seems equally damaging to endothelial cells in the small cerebral blood vessels. The Arginine Solution holds significant promise for restoring healthy levels of ADNO to the brain and, in so doing, enhancing its ability to function at its peak.

Forever Young: ADNO and the Aging Process

From Ponce de León's doomed quest for the fountain of youth to cutting-edge gerontological research at the National Institute on Aging, mankind has always held out the hope of staying young forever—or at least a bit longer. Little wonder, for the price of aging is considerable. Our skin wrinkles, our senses lose acuity, our reflexes and thought processes slow down. By the time we reach fifty most of us will have lost a full third of our lean muscle mass—replacing this, alas, with a surfeit of fat-storing adipose tissue. Our bones decalcify and lose density, predisposing us to fractures. The cardiovascular system becomes increasingly clogged and inflexible, exacerbating everything from hypertension to cognitive decline. No bodily system is exempt from deterioration. The digestive tract, for example, becomes sluggish and produces less stomach acid, leading to malabsorption of nutrients. The intestines and colon often erode in old age, triggering diverticular disease and painful rectal fissures called proctitis.

In women, the precipitous decline of estrogen at menopause causes a sudden jump in the risk of heart disease, depression, osteoporosis, and even Alzheimer's disease. In men, fluctuating levels of testosterone can fuel the growth of prostate tissue, which can cause urinary problems and possibly even prostate cancer. Most cancers, indeed, seem to surface first in middle age and later—the consequence, perhaps, of years of exposure to toxins and a gradual decline in the body's ability to protect itself.

In recent years, researchers have focused attention on a key hormone produced by the pituitary gland and known as HGH (human growth hormone). When we're young, HGH directs much of the growth process. It also oversees tissue repair throughout the body. Children are assured of a healthy HGH supply thanks to regular "bursts" of it released from the pituitary during sleep. By adolescence, these bursts occur during the day as well as at night. But with the growth spurt of our teenage years behind us, HGH production gradually wanes as we move ever deeper into adulthood. By the age of fifty, the pituitary of many people is releasing very slight amounts. By old age, fully half or more of adults are partially to totally deficient in HGH release. The key word here is "release"—for it turns out the pituitary does not lose its ability to produce HGH, just its ability to release what it stores.

In an article published in the *Journal of the American Geriatrics Society,* Dr. Daniel Rudman of the University of Chicago Medical School documented the many adverse changes that accompany aging, and speculated that these might, in part, be caused by HGH deficiency. Supplementation of this hormone in children with a deficiency had been used successfully to normalize growth. Might HGH supplements in the elderly serve as a rejuvenating "fountain of youth"?

In 1990, Dr. Rudman and his colleagues put this to a test in an important study subsequently published in *The New England Journal of Medicine.* They studied twenty-one otherwise healthy men, between the ages of sixty-one and eighty-seven, who suffered very low levels of HGH. One group then received an injection of synthetic HGH three times a week; the other group received no treatment. After six months, the men on HGH showed an 8.8 percent increase in lean muscle mass, a 14.4 percent decrease in fat tissue, a 1.6 percent increase in bone density, and a 7.1 percent increase in skin thickness. On these measures, at least, HGH clearly proved rejuvenating. The men who didn't receive HGH, on the other hand, showed none of these beneficial changes.[12]

Injection of such a potent hormone is not free of significant side effects. The good news is that you may not need to receive weekly injections to derive these same benefits. In research dating back to the 1960s, arginine was shown to be an effective way to boost HGH. Indeed, an article in *The Lancet* found that intravenous infusion of thirty grams of arginine led to an astonishing 1,100 percent increase in HGH in healthy women.[13] A follow-up study in *The New England Journal of Medicine* reported that such infusion "was entirely without side effects in a large personal experience."

But because infusion is not a practical delivery system for most individuals, other researchers have sought to determine an effective oral dose. In one small study, men aged twenty to thirty-five were given approximately seventeen grams of oral L-arginine per day for a week. This led to a 58 percent increase in the release of nighttime HGH. Of course, seventeen grams per day is several times more than the three to six grams we recommend. Will our lower-dose Arginine Solution still impact HGH? Though no studies, to our knowledge, have yet been performed to answer this question, we suspect many people will have at least a modest increase in HGH. In a way, a small change may actually be preferable to a more dramatic one, especially in the light of recent question marks surrounding the possible effects of HGH on some cancer-cell growth. (For more on this, see Chapter 14.)

Also unclear at this point is the role arginine-stimulated HGH can play in weight loss. Dietary supplements of arginine inhibit fat absorption and lower cholesterol in addition to promoting HGH release.[14] In light of HGH's ability to build muscle mass and decrease body fat, researchers began to wonder if arginine supplements might prove therapeutic in the treatment of obesity. Scientists at the University of California at San Francisco gave thirty grams of arginine daily by injection to ten healthy and ten obese patients. The good news for the healthy volunteers was that arginine triggered a six-fold rise in HGH release. The not-so-good news for the obese volunteers was that they enjoyed only a tiny rise, leading the authors to conclude that arginine is unlikely to play much of a role, if any, in the treatment of obesity.[15]

What we can say with certainty, however, is that arginine can benefit one of the most important, age-related physiological declines: the damage to blood vessels, which itself serves as the first tilted domino in so many deleterious chain reactions. As Dr. Anoop Chauhan put it, in the December 7, 1995, internist and cardiologist edition of the *Medical Tribune,* "We have demonstrated for the first time that you can reverse this [aging] effect with L-arginine."[16]

The Arginine Solution gives new meaning to the phrase "young at heart."

Mother and Child

There is a unique form of hypertension called preeclampsia that affects an estimated 7 to 10 percent of pregnant women, usually but not always during a first pregnancy. Symptoms generally develop in the final trimester and usually feature dangerously elevated blood pressure, fluid retention that leads to swollen hands and feet and a puffy face, and elevated levels of protein in the urine. In severe cases, the condition can evolve into life-threatening eclampsia itself or a variant form called HELLP syndrome. Without treatment, women can suffer convulsions, coma, and death. Indeed, in the United States, Great Britain, and Scandinavia, preeclampsia is the leading cause of death for mothers and infants alike in the moments right after childbirth. Fortunately, for most women, delivery brings a speedy return to normal blood pressure.

What triggers preeclampsia remains mysterious, but clues now point to a failure of nitric oxide production. Blood volume during pregnancy increases by up to 40 percent. You might expect this to heighten blood pressure in almost anyone. After all, if you force a lot of extra water into your garden hose, pressure has to go up, right?

In garden hoses, yes. In healthy pregnant women, no. Blood pressure actually stays more or less the same, and may even fall a little, despite the addition of so much blood. The reason: A large increase in NO made from arginine greatly expands the diameter of blood vessels, providing ample room for extra blood. Women with preeclampsia, on the other hand, don't seem to enjoy this beneficial elevation of NO or the consequent dilation; thus their blood pressure rises.[17]

But what about nitric oxide and the developing fetus? In 1991, researchers from the University of Cincinnati College of Medicine showed that the placenta can generate nitric oxide, which then acts to dilate the blood vessels of the fetus, thus promoting an adequate blood supply.[18]

Women suffering preeclampsia are sometimes given magnesium injections to reduce not only blood pressure but also muscle spasms and seizures. Such treatment is usually effective, but not always. To date, there have been no human trials of arginine therapy, but in lab animals stimulated to develop preeclamptic symptoms, arginine normalized blood pressure and reduced the amount of protein in urine.[19]

At least one human case study was recently reported in *The Lancet.* This involved a forty-one-year-old expectant mother from London who was admitted to the hospital during the thirty-eighth week of her second pregnancy. The reason for admission: Her blood pressure was dangerously high—200/95 mm HG—and her blood and urine alike carried abnormal levels of protein. The same day, she gave birth to a healthy baby girl. Most of the time, the mother's blood pressure quickly stabilizes, but this time it remained dangerously high long after the birth. Her doctors gave her conventional treatment, including intravenous magnesium, but she went on to suffer two convulsions.[20]

It was at this point that the doctors decided to try an intravenous infusion of a substance that, like arginine, the body can use to make nitric oxide. After about an hour of steady infusion, the woman's blood pressure had lowered to the normal range. She and her baby have been thriving ever since.

Does the Arginine Solution hold promise for treating preeclampsia in the future? It's too early to know for sure, but researchers are encouraged by the work done to date. The same holds true for ADNO and the prevention of premature labor and preterm birth. Obstetricians have long observed a correlation between strong "spontaneous" contractions of the uterus and a woman's risk of delivering her child early. A recent article in the *American Journal of Obstetrics and Gynecology* reported that nitric oxide derived from arginine seems to inhibit these contractions and maintain uterine quiescence.[21]

Does this mean that pregnant women should take arginine supplements? Though some researchers believe the Arginine Solution might one day emerge as a logical treatment and/or preventative measure for preeclampsia and preterm labor alike, it's still too early to know for sure. Our best advice: Stay tuned.

Opening the Lungs

Asthma refers to a group of related diseases caused by constriction of the breathing passages of the lungs. Fluid then frequently accumulates in the little terminal bronchial sacs, leading to inflammation and a further reduction in a victim's ability to take in a refreshing breath of air. Asthma can run the gamut from the barely noticeable to the sometimes fatal. A variety of triggers, including such allergens as those in pollen, pollution, and even cockroach shells, have been proposed as contributing factors in asthma attacks. Whatever the causes, cases of asthma and fatalities from it have climbed alarmingly in recent years, particularly in inner cities. Regardless of what precipitates an episode, researchers at the National Heart and Lung Institute in England showed for the first time that the mechanism that keeps bronchial passages open in the lungs is controlled entirely by nitric oxide.[22]

A thoracic specialist at the institute gave volunteers dosages of arginine that ranged from 3.4 grams to 13.6 grams daily. The higher the dosage of arginine, the greater the increase in nitric oxide in exhaled breath. All but one of the volunteers receiving arginine showed signs of improved lung function. Volunteers on placebos showed no changes.

Increasing nitric oxide available to the lungs via inhalers has become an accepted therapy for a number of more severe lung-related diseases, including adult respiratory distress syndrome, pulmonary hypertension, and chronic obstructive pulmonary disease.[23] This latter condition, often abbreviated COPD, is the fourth leading cause of death in the United States, killing more people each year than AIDS, suicide, and liver diseases put together.

Will the Arginine Solution help you if you suffer from asthma or other lung diseases? Studies to date are promising but not definitive. Talk it over with your doctor before giving it a try.

Stopping a Real Pain in the Butt

If you've ever suffered from hemorrhoids or an anal fissure, you'll never again be able to take the phrase "pain in the butt" lightly. As victims well know, these conditions cause a host of maddening symptoms that range from itching and pain to rectal bleeding and spasms of the anal sphincter muscles.

Doctors now know that it is a chronic contraction of these internal sphincter muscles that likely causes hemorrhoids and fissures in the first place. Moreover, researchers at Oxford University Medical College recently discovered that nitric oxide is the chemical signaler that instructs these muscles to relax. When they gave volunteers a formulation to inhibit the enzyme that makes nitric oxide synthase, the muscles clenched down. When they subsequently provided arginine, the muscles relaxed.[24]

To see if this mechanism might be applied therapeutically, Dr. Stephen R. Gorfine at the Mount Sinai School of Medicine tried giving patients suffering external hemorrhoids or anal fissures a topically applied ointment containing nitroglycerin. This substance, like arginine, increases the supply of available NO.[25]

At first, most patients reported pain relief that lasted two to six hours following application. Within two weeks, ten of the patients had healed completely. Two others were symptom-free within a month. The anal lesions persisted longer in the remaining patients, but all were pain-free.

Subsequent studies in *The New England Journal of Medicine,* *The Lancet,* and the *British Journal of Surgery* all confirmed the effectiveness of such treatment.[26, 27, 28] To date, however, no studies have been done to show whether the Arginine Solution can help prevent these "pains in the butt" by boosting available NO supply through oral supplementation of arginine. In theory, at least, the possibility definitely seems promising enough to warrant further investigation.

Sickle Cell Disease

Sickle cell disease is an inherited condition characterized by abnormalities in hemoglobin, which, in turn, cause the red blood cells that contain it to become crescent-shaped instead of round, usually resulting in anemia. In areas of the world such as Africa where malaria is common and frequently deadly, sickle cell disease seems to be less a "disease" than a survival strategy. The parasites that cause malaria have trouble penetrating these odd-shaped blood cells. What's more, changes in the blood cell membrane permeability encourage the influx of potassium, a chemical the parasites find decidedly unpalatable.

Such benefits, though not inconsiderable if you contract malaria, nonetheless come with a hefty price tag. Victims of sickle cell disease can suffer sluggish circulation, which can result in fatigue, dizzy spells, rapid heartbeat, greater susceptibility to pneumonia and other infections, severe joint pain, and eventually major organ damage and failure.

Since the landmark discovery of NO's role in hemoglobin was first made by Dr. Jonathan S. Stamler and his colleagues at Duke University Medical Center, sickle cell experts have begun focusing on nitric oxide as a way of ensuring that small blood vessels stay open and don't become clogged by the crescent-shaped cells. Such clogging is known to trigger inflammation and cause the crippling joint pain seen in some sickle cell patients.[29]

The researchers concluded that the crisis in the sickle cell disease may have been brought about by the failure of nitric oxide production leading to blood-vessel constriction and obstruction. In an interview with *The New York Times,* Dr. Stamler sounded a cautionary note: "It makes sense to give nitric oxide and oxygen to people with this disease, but we first have to do more research to look at the consequences of such an approach." In this, he is proposing the inhalation of nitric oxide, a therapeutic approach that has already been used to treat patients with pulmonary hypertension and respiratory distress syndrome successfully.

As of the date of this book's publication, we're unaware of any published reports on oral arginine as a way of combating sickle cell disease. The field of ADNO research, however, continues to explode on many levels. We're confident it's only a brief matter of time before the logic of the Arginine Solution for sickle cell disease is tested in clinical trials.

Nitric oxide is such a ubiquitous and important substance in the human body that at least one top researcher has declared, "It does everything, everywhere!" Indeed, a host of seemingly unrelated miscellaneous health problems, from Alzheimer's disease to diabetes to hemorrhoids, all seem to have one thing in common: They're caused or exacerbated by a deficiency of nitric oxide.

Researchers searching for ways to treat and prevent these disorders have begun to investigate the use of arginine, via injection or oral supplements, as a way to boost NO levels and benefit patients. Such benefits can occur through several different processes that NO regulates. For instance, NO-mediated dilation of blood vessels keeps oxygen and glucose flowing freely to the brain, thus preventing the cognitive decline that hypoxia can cause. NO also serves as a neurotransmitter that allows nerve cells to communicate even when they aren't directly connected.

Among other effects, NO from arginine may also promote the release of insulin, which could benefit diabetics, and human growth hormone (HGH), which improves body composition and may play a role in retarding the aging process.

Because many of ADNO's multiple effects have only so recently been discovered, the potential worth of arginine supplements for treating many conditions has not yet been explored in clinical trials. The evidence that has been collected, however, remains highly promising. In the coming years, we are confident that the Arginine Solution will be a well-validated and widespread staple of preventative and complementary health care for a wide variety of medical conditions.

14

Know When to Say No
A Few Cautions on the Use of ADNO

First, do no harm.
—Hippocrates

There is no substance on earth, no matter how beneficial its effects, that does not simultaneously contain within it the ability to harm. Take oxygen, for instance, the sine qua non of our existence. When deprived of this molecule for more than a few minutes, our brain cells begin to die in droves, and our other body tissues soon follow suit.

But as doctors treating premature infants in the 1950s discovered, too much of a good thing can sometimes pose its own set of problems. Infants whose lungs were not fully developed at birth were routinely administered nearly pure oxygen in the belief that this would help boost blood-oxygen levels quickly and enhance their survival odds. Many of these preemies did, indeed, survive because of it, but such concentrated oxygen damaged their retinas and left a high percentage partly to completely blinded for life. Today, neonatal specialists have learned to provide their tiniest patients with lower concentrations of oxygen, which prevents this tragic side effect.

The next time you're in a drugstore, take a look at the fine print accompanying even the most innocuous of over-the-counter drugs. The list of contraindications—i.e., reasons why certain patients should avoid the remedy—is shocking. Ordinary calcium antacids, for example, can threaten the lives of people suffering impaired kidney function. Tylenol, especially when consumed with too much alcohol, can cause catastrophic liver damage that has resulted in convulsions, coma, and even death. The decongestants found in cold remedies can jack up blood pressure and even trigger hallucinations and seizures in susceptible individuals. Even consuming too much water can hurt you—a rare syndrome called psychogenic water drinking leaves victims with a dangerous imbalance in their blood chemistry.

If you are looking for an absolutely 100 percent safe substance, you will not find it in your pharmacy. Nor, for that matter, will you find it in a grocery store—or even in nature itself.

Our point in bringing all this up is not to unduly alarm you with the widely held canard: Everything can kill you! It is to alert you to the fact that when you take any substance, from nutritional supplements to drugs, you should be aware of the relative risks and benefits. It is our way of acknowledging that some of the same biochemical properties that make ADNO so beneficial to a host of bodily systems *may* (and we emphasize *may*) make it inappropriate if you have certain medical conditions.

In reviewing research reports currently available in medical libraries, we have come across a handful of such conditions, which we will be presenting shortly. In most cases, any adverse effect of ADNO remains more theoretical than proven. Moreover, the dosage levels that triggered any deleterious effects, when such occurred, were usually the result of arginine infusion at much higher dosage levels (usually thirty to fifty grams given intravenously) than the relatively modest three to six grams of oral supplements we've consistently recommended.

Nowhere in the literature did we find the suggestion that any patient, suffering from any condition, should avoid the arginine naturally found in his or her diet. That our Arginine Solution represents at most a doubling of the normal dietary intake further adds to our confidence that it is safe for most individuals who begin a daily regimen.

ADNO research, to be sure, continues apace around the globe. In coming years, medical practitioners will no doubt have a much better grasp of how to tailor supplemental ADNO therapy to the specific needs of different patients. For now, if you do suffer from one of the conditions listed below, you *must* consult your doctor before initiating arginine supplementation.

If he or she is unfamiliar with ADNO, this book and the studies cited in it will likely prove both useful and illuminating. Moreover, because the latest discoveries on ADNO's effects usually appear in professional journals first, your doctor would have had a chance to learn about new therapeutic applications—and contraindications—long before these filter down to general-interest publications or the broadcast media.

It also just makes good sense to keep your partner in health care fully informed about any steps you are taking to keep yourself well. That way, he or she can better see the whole picture—and tailor other treatments, when needed, accordingly.

Just as important, we ask that you also consult *yourself*. Listen to your body, pay attention to its signals, for you should know it better than any "experts" possibly can. This is not to say you should try to self-diagnose every potential disorder. Sometimes silent changes occur—and sometimes, through neglect or denial, we minimize odd symptoms in the hopes that they'll simply disappear. This is one reason why the partnership between doctor and patient is so critical.

If supplemental arginine does not agree with your system, if you find that it provokes side effects or even a subtle sense of unease, then cut back on the dosage, or eliminate it entirely. Each individual is unique, and no two people ever respond exactly the same to any treatment. In our own practices, we have not yet seen any significant adverse reactions, but we remain open to their possibility. It is for this reason that we reiterate: Listen to your body and follow the advice it sounds.

For the overwhelming majority of you, we're confident you'll like what you hear. Indeed, we suspect that for many of you arginine supplements will, over time, lead you to a gradual but steady recognition that your overall health is improving; to a sense of improved cardiovascular functioning; to perhaps an immune system that is staving off infections with a renewed vigor; even your sexuality and cognitive abilities are operating nearer the top of their respective games. We have seen such changes in our patients and in ourselves, just as we have witnessed firsthand the bolstered psychological sense of well-being that accompanies these positive improvements in physical health. For many individuals, the Arginine Solution can help initiate an upward spiral that will carry the body and the mind toward a healthier place.

The same may apply as well to people who have been diagnosed with the following disorders. However, enough question marks still remain about nitric oxide's complex roles in these conditions that we would be remiss if we did not add a few cautionary notes where needed. The bottom line: If you have a history of one or more of these ailments, or you know that you are at high risk for developing one, consult with your doctor before taking arginine supplements.

Migraines

Derived from the French word *megrim* ("morbid low spirits") and the Greek words *hemi crania* (literally "half the head"), a migraine typically produces a severe headache on one side of a sufferer's head and assorted other symptoms that can include tunnel vision, scintillating light patterns in the visual field, sensitivity to light, dizziness, nausea, runny nose, coldness in the extremities, and many other peculiar effects. Not every victim suffers all of these, of course—indeed it's possible to have a migraine attack without even enduring a headache at all. Most patients, alas, aren't so lucky. An often excruciating headache builds in intensity just as the visual disturbances begin subsiding. The resulting pain can persist for as little as a few hours, or as long as several days.

If you get migraines, chances are you had your first attack in your youth. Sixty percent of sufferers have an initial onset before the age of sixteen, and 90 percent have their first migraine before forty. Late-onset migraines are not unheard of, but they're very rare. If you've so far made it into middle age unscathed, chances are good this is one health problem you won't need to worry about in the future.

The exact cause of migraines has only recently begun yielding its secrets to scientific investigators. As far back as the late 1920s, researchers noted an abnormal pattern of blood-vessel activity in the heads of migraine sufferers. This begins with spasmodic contractions of the arteries, followed by an "overkill" vessel dilation. The headache pain appears to be a direct result of the rapid dilation phase. Drugs like beta-blockers, which prevent vessel constriction in the first place, are sometimes used to nip the whole process in the bud. Without an initial spasmodic contraction, the arteries don't dilate. Hence no migraine.

The question for researchers has long been: What intrinsic factors trigger these blood vessel changes? One theory championed by British neurologist Dr. E. Hanington has to do with the tendency of blood platelets to clump together.[1] Relatively high levels of the ubiquitous neurotransmitter serotonin can cause this aggregation in most people. Hanington suggested that migraine sufferers may have an inherited abnormality that allows much lower levels of serotonin than normal to trigger platelet clumping. The rapid dilation of arterioles may be the body's self-protective reaction to this clumping, or it may result from more direct effects of serotonin on vessel walls. In any event, new-generation migraine drugs like sumatriptan (brand name: Imitrex), when delivered by injection or orally, can bring dramatic and speedy relief by directly blocking serotonin.

But is serotonin the only substance implicated in the migraine process? More recent research suggests that it may not be. In 1997, a Danish research group published a paper in *The Lancet* suggesting that one of the body's other potent vasodilators—nitric oxide—may also play a role in causing and/or sustaining attacks.[2] As evidence for this, the researchers gave fifteen migraine patients a drug that inhibits the enzyme that makes NO from arginine. Two-thirds of the patients enjoyed significant relief from their symptoms, compared to only 25 percent on placebo. The researchers' conclusion: "Inhibiting NO production or reducing the effects of NO may therefore represent a completely novel therapeutic principle in migraine."

Many questions, to be sure, remain about this so-called nitric oxide hypothesis of migraine, and the case is far from proven. Given the uncertainties, however, it seems only prudent to avoid arginine supplementation directly preceding, or during, a migraine attack. Moreover, if you are a frequent migraine sufferer and you find that daily arginine supplements are adversely impacting the frequency or intensity of attacks, discuss the regimen with your physician before continuing supplementation.

Depression

Theories about the cause of depression have ranged from evil demons burrowing inside the skull to the equally unsubstantiated psychoanalytic myth that it represents anger turned inward, to more modern notions that stress the impact of pessimistic thinking and other cognitive distortions on self-perception and thus mood. More and more researchers, however, are concluding that the root cause of depression often has a decidedly more concrete basis: an imbalance of neurotransmitter substances in the brain. Antidepressant medications, which can eliminate depressive symptoms in many patients after years of "talk therapy" have failed, lend support to the idea that depression is, in many cases, a case of brain chemistry gone awry.

One of the neurotransmitters most closely linked to depression is serotonin, an extremely complex chemical found at numerous sites throughout the body, from the brain to the gut, each sporting its own subtype of serotonin receptor cell. Depending on the location, serotonin can exert a multitude of different effects. Of keenest interest to those in a depression, of course, is serotonin's effect in the brain. Here, when present in sufficient quantities, it appears to promote feelings of well-being, warding off anxiety and depression. A host of new-generation antidepressant medications called SSRIs (for selective serotonin reuptake inhibitors) make use of this fact. They work not by causing the brain to produce extra serotonin, but rather by keeping the serotonin it does produce available longer.

But serotonin may have another effect in the brain as well, one that could warrant caution in taking arginine supplements for those who are prone to clinical depression. Cardiologists at the University of Pittsburgh School of Medicine recently reported that serotonin levels and nitric oxide production may both be linked in depression. They noted that the antidepressant drug paroxetine (Paxil, a close chemical cousin of the famous fluoxetine, aka Prozac) not only boosted levels of serotonin in patients' brains, but it also appeared to reduce levels of NO, which itself can serve as a neurotransmitter. The fact that both results paralleled improvement in depressive symptoms raises the possibility, at least in theory, that too much ADNO in susceptible individuals can compound mood disturbances.[3]

If you are taking arginine supplements and are prone to depression, our best advice is to be vigilant about any adverse impact on your mood. Future research may well find that the NO link to depression is a red herring, but until more is known, it makes sense to remain alert to a possible connection.

The same advice also likely applies to individuals who suffer from a rare weather sensitivity known as the serotonin irritation syndrome. You may have heard the phrase coined by English epigrammatist John Heywood: "It's an ill wind that blows no good." In susceptible individuals, this "ill wind" is more than just a metaphor. Indeed, dry desert winds variously known as mistrals in France, siroccos in Italy, sharavs in Israel, chinooks in the Rocky Mountains, and Santa Ana winds in southern California have all been shown to impact the health and mood of certain people adversely, triggering symptoms that can range from dizziness and fatigue to headaches and depression. As far back as 1958, researchers showed that the positively charged air ions that are a hallmark of these "ill winds" can increase breathing rate and blood pressure in up to 25 percent of the population.[4]

The likely mechanism, according to work done at the U.S. Naval Biological Laboratory, is that the positive ions somehow increase serotonin, which then leads to a corresponding boost in NO production.[5] Why *increasing* levels of serotonin and NO would accompany depression and hypertension remains paradoxical. What has been demonstrated, however, is that drugs that either directly or indirectly block NO production seem to be helpful in controlling the unpleasant symptoms that accompany serotonin irritation syndrome. Again, until more is known, if your mood tends to plummet when an ill wind blows, it may make sense to avoid boosting ADNO till calm is restored.

Autoimmune Disorders

As you saw in Chapter 12, ADNO can be one of your immune system's greatest allies because it provides macrophages and other immune cells with the powerful nitric oxide "bullets" they need to kill invaders, suppress cancers, and bollix up the DNA replication of the body's internal enemies. In a sense, you can think of ADNO as the body's armamentarium, the place immune cells go when they need more ammo to fight the enemy.

In autoimmune diseases, however, it is as if the immune system somehow loses its ability to perceive our own body parts as separate from the enemy and thus begins raining "friendly fire" on some of the same tissues it's supposed to protect. No one knows for sure how the immune system becomes so confused. One theory suggests that an infectious agent, such as a virus or bacteria, provokes the initial attack, which continues long after the microbe has been vanquished.

Regardless of the mechanism behind autoimmune problems, the last thing you would want to give your body when it's begun attacking itself is more bullets. This makes theoretical sense, but does it apply in real patients? Consider the evidence for such a conclusion in a handful of relatively common autoimmune disorders.

Ulcerative colitis, Crohn's disease, and related inflammatory bowel disease afflict some 150,000 Americans per year. Symptoms can range from low-grade intestinal upset to bloody diarrhea and joint pain. In particularly nasty cases, the digestive system can become so inflamed that it impairs the absorption of nutrients, leading to anemia and starvation.

Theories for what initiates the inflammation range from genetic susceptibility to food allergy to gastrointestinal bacteria. In coming years, these diseases may yield to a combination of antibiotic and anti-inflammatory drug treatment, but for now they remain largely incurable. Once the immune system begins its self-attack, it is often exceedingly difficult to call a truce.

The nitric oxide link to inflammatory bowel diseases first began to emerge in 1993 when medical researchers at the Wellcome Laboratories and the University Hospital in Nottingham, England, reported that patients with ulcerative colitis had greatly increased levels of the enzyme that macrophages and lymphocytes use to make NO.[6] In 1994, a Swedish research team demonstrated that patients with ulcerative colitis were making *100 times* more NO than normal in the lining of their colons.[7] As evidence continued to accumulate that these astronomical levels of NO might be responsible for the lesions and other harmful changes in the lining of the colon, as opposed to an attempt to heal the inflammation, it was only a matter of time before investigators would try inactivating the NO enzyme to see if this would positively impact a patient's condition. In 1995, medical researchers from the department of medicine and pathology at McMasters University in Canada found exactly this positive effect—in rats.[8] As of this writing, we have found no similar studies in humans. For the moment, however, we recommend against arginine supplementation in any patient with inflammatory bowel disease.

Another common autoimmune disorder, rheumatoid arthritis, is characterized by often severe joint pain. Most patients develop it after the age of forty, though a different form, called Still's disease, or juvenile rheumatoid arthritis, can occur in kids as young as two years old. Women are two to three times more likely than men to develop either form. Women are indeed much more vulnerable than men to most autoimmune diseases.

As with ulcerative colitis, researchers have known for a while that inhibiting the enzyme that macrophages use to produce nitric oxide can reduce joint inflammation in rodents. In 1994, two researchers from the department of pharmacology at King's College, in London, set about to determine if such nitric oxide-mediated damage also occurs in human inflammatory joint disease. Among other findings, they determined that the fluid in inflamed human joints did indeed contain elevated levels of this same enzyme.[9] But what does all this mean for arginine supplementation?

Though human testing has not yet been done, one study of rats with rheumatoid arthritis sounds a distinctly cautionary note. As reported in the *British Journal of Pharmacology*, test animals were assigned to one of three groups. The first received arginine in their drinking water. The second was given an inhibitor of the nitric oxide enzyme. And the third received plain water.

Those receiving arginine showed significant swelling in arthritic paws, whereas those who got the inhibiting agent actually enjoyed a reduction in swelling. The effect was strong enough that the researchers concluded with the suggestion that powerful anti-inflammatory drugs, like prednisone, may work in part by impairing nitric oxide production. Though these findings remain preliminary, we strongly urge individuals with rheumatoid arthritis to avoid supplemental arginine until more is known. It may be especially important not to supplement with arginine while also taking cortisone.

One other disease thought to be at least partly autoimmune is multiple sclerosis, a malady with particularly devastating consequences to young adults. Striking roughly twice as many women as men and twice as many whites as blacks, MS affects the fatty myelin sheath that surrounds certain nerve fibers like the insulation on household wires. For reasons that are not yet understood, the immune system of MS victims begins attacking this sheath in the spine and brain, replacing healthy insulation with an abnormal form of plaque. Doctors now recognize four distinct versions of the disease that range in intensity from the so-called benign form, which causes temporary symptoms that eventually go into permanent remission, to the so-called chronic-progressive form of MS, which can leave victims incontinent, blind, and wheelchair bound.

In 1995, British scientists first implicated excessive NO production in multiple sclerosis, showing significantly elevated levels of NO markers in the spinal fluid of MS patients over what they found in healthy people.[10] Follow-up work in 1997 reconfirmed this finding, and showed that AIDS patients revealed similar elevations in NO.[11] The authors' conclusion: Drugs that inhibit NO synthesis may have some value in treating these diseases. Therefore, in neurodegenerative diseases such MS, arginine supplementation should not be done without the advice of a knowledgeable physician.

Other Caveats

We found only a few other health problems for which the Arginine Solution is at least theoretically contraindicated. High doses of arginine, in the range of thirty grams or more infused directly into the bloodstream, very rarely cause significant side effects.

AIDS research is incredibly complex, and results are rarely definitive. Case in point: By 1993, different teams had concluded that NO's antiviral properties might at once help and hurt AIDS patients. NO may benefit them by helping destroy the HIV virus. It conceivably hurts them when hyperactive "NO-shooting" macrophages attack HIV inside brain cells, sort of like G-men of old who end up destroying a house to get at the crooks hiding inside. The researchers suggested that inflammation and other resulting nerve damage from the NO attack may be a prime cause of AIDS-related dementia. As is the case with autoimmune disorders as well, NO appears for some patients to be a two-edged sword. Again, till the exact mechanisms involved are better understood, arginine supplements should probably be avoided by people who have AIDS—and perhaps also by those who are HIV-positive without AIDS.

Arginine has been shown to help successfully combat many cancers, but when it comes to **breast cancer,** the jury is still out. As far back as 1981, the National Cancer Institute reported that arginine-derived nitric oxide inhibits breast-cancer-cell replication in a test tube.[12, 13] Other studies showed the same effect in living animals.[14] But in 1992, another team reported that in humans, arginine can have paradoxical effects. On the one hand, arginine definitely stimulates the immune-system cells that battle breast cancer, providing macrophages with the bullets to kill tumor cells and inhibit their reproduction.[15]

On the other hand, arginine also seems to stimulate tumor growth in breast cancer patients, at least when administered in high daily doses of thirty to fifty grams. No one knows for sure what, if any, mechanism is at work here. It may be that arginine works either as a nutrient or as a human growth hormone (HGH) releaser.

Ironically, this greater proliferation of tumor cells has a silver lining. Researchers have actually found that because of their rapid replication, tumor cells are more easily killed by chemotherapy. For this reason, it's likely that arginine may one day play an important role in treating the disease. Until more is known, however, women with breast cancer—or those who are at high risk for the disease—should refrain from dietary arginine supplementation, even at modest doses.

This said, however, it is important also to bear in mind that arginine has never been shown to *cause* breast cancer. All cells have nutrient requirements, and it may turn out that certain breast cancers might require additional arginine. This would hardly be a unique finding. An August 1997 National Cancer Institute study, for instance, showed that common polyunsaturated vegetable oil, such as corn or safflower oil, enhanced the growth of cancer cells in living tissues. In terms of arginine, it is reassuring to note that the only time such an adverse reaction has been demonstrated was in women with advanced breast cancer who received clinical dosages of thirty to fifty grams intravenously—not the conservative oral dosages of three to six grams per day.

The good news is that, to date, no connection between ordinary oral arginine supplementation and any other form of cancer has been reported. Indeed, as discussed in Chapter 12, arginine often inhibits the growth of many types of cancer.

Cirrhosis is an irreversible progressive degenerative liver disease that may result from a number of different causes. Alcohol and its attendant vitamin and other nutritional deficiencies and hepatitis are the most common of these. Cirrhosis can cause impaired protein synthesis and elevated blood ammonia levels. It is often characterized by a discoloration of the skin, which we call jaundice.

Recent studies have shown that persons with liver cirrhosis show elevated exhaled NO.[16] A recent report in the *Annals of Internal Medicine* tells us that in those cases where a liver transplant was required and successful, exhaled nitric oxide subsequently decreased, suggesting that nitric oxide is an important mediator of impaired oxygenation in patients with cirrhosis.[17] Yet another recent report, in *The New England Journal of Medicine*, likewise cautions that increased nitric oxide production in cirrhosis may contribute to a low blood pressure complication in advanced disease.[18] Consequently, we presently advise against arginine supplementation in persons with this disease.

Hyperkalemia, or extremely high levels of potassium in the blood, has been reported in patients with existing kidney disease as well as in two men suffering from chronic alcoholism. If you are generally healthy and stick to the modest three to six grams of oral arginine we recommend, the risk of developing hyperkalemia is low. On the other hand, if you are on medication known to affect potassium levels, such as aldactone or ACE inhibitors, or if you are a very heavy drinker of alcohol or have impaired kidney function, consult with your doctor about arginine's possible effects on potassium levels.

Another condition where nitric oxide may play an adverse role is in **septic shock,** commonly called blood poisoning. In response to a massive infection, the body rallies by producing an equally massive outpouring of nitric oxide. On the plus side, this arms macrophages with the bullets they need to fight the invading germs, and it also selectively relaxes blood vessels so as to redistribute blood flow where it's most necessary. On the negative side, however, this vasodilation can sometimes go too far, causing blood pressure throughout the body to drop to dangerously low levels. In 1996, investigators reported in the *Journal of the American Medical Association* that giving septic-shock patients medication that inhibits NO formation can raise blood pressure safely and save lives.[19] Obviously, arginine should not be given to such patients.

Although it has been shown in previous chapters that arginine can prevent **stroke** through lower blood pressure, lower cholesterol, and reduced platelet aggregation, too much NO during and immediately following a stroke may be dangerous and actually increase brain-cell death. In animal models in which a stroke was simulated by choking off a brain artery, blocking NO synthesis has been shown to limit the extent of brain damage. For this reason, supplemental arginine should *not* be given to someone immediately after suffering a stroke, nor to individuals who are at high risk of suffering a stroke. Bear in mind that NO is harmful only *after* a stroke has occurred. For most individuals, regular arginine supplements can *reduce* the risk of this happening.

Most knowledgeable authorities also recommend that one not take an arginine supplement during an active **herpes** or herpes zoster infection because it can interfere with the action of another amino acid, lysine, which is one of the body's most effective herpes virus hunters.

You should likewise exercise caution if you are currently taking the anti-impotence medication **Viagra** (sildenafil citrate), and/or **NO donors** like nitroglycerin. Like arginine supplements themselves, all these drugs work in varying ways to increase blood-vessel dilation. The combination of L-arginine along with one or more of these other drugs can conceivably open your blood vessels too much, leading to dangerously low blood pressure.

It is probably only a matter of time before it becomes public knowledge that arginine may often be a safer substitute for Viagra. We caution that you consult with your physician about the safety of arginine supplementation in conjunction with Viagra.

The Arginine Solution is a safe and effective form of complementary care for a wide array of common health problems, from disorders of the heart and circulatory system to a lackluster immune response. The same qualities that make ADNO so beneficial, however, may—in some instances—also cause problems. For example, the dilation of blood vessels that is so helpful in controlling hypertension can, theoretically, also dilate blood vessels in the head of a migraine sufferer, sustaining the misery of an attack. Likewise, the powerful NO bullets that macrophages use to kill invading microbes, when turned against the body itself as appears to be the case in autoimmune diseases, may injure and sometimes even destroy vital tissues.

Other diseases as well, from stroke to septic shock, can both benefit from increased nitric oxide and be exacerbated by it. In these cases, the jury is still out on whether these benefits outweigh the drawbacks, or vice versa. What's more, no researcher can yet begin to quantify a dose level of arginine above which problems are most likely to occur, if indeed they even do. It definitely bears repeating that when very high experimental doses of arginine—thirty to fifty grams or more—were directly infused into the bloodstream of study volunteers, rarely did anyone report any significant side effects. Certainly, we are not aware of any problems in our own patients who follow the conservative regimen we recommend, i.e., three to six grams taken daily by mouth.

For those suffering from one of the contraindicated conditions discussed in this chapter, it's important to discuss arginine supplementation with your doctor first. For the millions of other men and women hoping to stay in top health—or just hoping to move closer in that direction—consider the words of Hippocrates himself, who said, "Healing is a matter of time, but it is sometimes also a matter of opportunity." (The reader should bear in mind that no long-term studies have been reported, but at the relatively low doses recommended for this nutrient, it is unlikely that it would produce harmful side effects.)

In the twilight of the twentieth century, medical researchers have provided us all with an exceptional new opportunity. And for those capable of availing themselves of it, the Arginine Solution promises to be a true and forceful ally in the quest for good health.

Appendix

Arginine and arginine-based products are distributed by several nutraceutical firms, such as:

- Real Health Laboratories, San Diego, CA (800) 565-6656
- Takeda America, Orangeburg, NY (800) 825-3328
- Schweizerhall, Piscataway, NJ (908) 981-8200
- Ajinomoto USA, Teaneck, NJ (201) 907-3225
- DNP International, Terre Haute, IN (812) 232-2211
- Stauber Performance, Brea, CA (714) 990-6663
- Kyowa Hakko, USA Inc., Newport Beach, CA (949) 833-0141

You should discuss your choice of products with your physician and consider such guidelines as the following:

- Each compound in a given formula should have scientific substantiation for its inclusion, supported by references in reputable conventional scientific and clinical publications.
- Products should be manufactured in an FDA-registered, pharmaceutically licensed facility.
- Products should only be composed of USP-grade materials, where applicable.
- Quality and potency of the finished products should be validated through analytical testing by an independent AOAC laboratory, and evidence to that effect should be available upon request.

REFERENCES

CHAPTER 2

1. Stamler, J. S., Jia, L., Eu, J. P., McMahon, T. J., Demchenko, I. T., Bonaventura, J., Gerbert, K., and Piantadosi, C. A., "Blood Flow Regulation by S-Nitrosohemoglobin in the Physiological Oxygen Gradient," *Science,* 276 (1997), 2034–2036.

CHAPTER 3

1. McCully, K. S., *The Homocysteine Revolution* (New Canaan, Ct.: Keats Publishing Inc., 1997).
2. Koshland, D. E., "The Molecule of the Year," *Science,* 258 (1992), 1861–1863.
3. Joint National Committee, "The 1988 Report of the Joint National Committee on Detection, Evaluation, and Treatment of High Blood Pressure," *Archives of Internal Medicine,* 148, 1023–1038.
4. Ornish, D. M., *Dr. Dean Ornish's Program for Reversing Heart Disease* (New York: Random House, 1990).

CHAPTER 4

1. Stamler, J. S., Jia, L., Eu, J. P., McMahon, T. J., Demchenko, I. T., Bonaventura, J., Gerbert, K., and Piantadosi, C. A., "Blood Flow Regulation by S-Nitrosohemoglobin in the Physiological Oxygen Gradient," *Science,* 276 (1997), 2034–2036.
2. Ornish, D. M., *Dr. Dean Ornish's Program for Reversing Heart Disease* (New York: Random House, 1990).
3. Blakeslee, S., "Surprise Discovery in Blood: Hemoglobin Has Bigger Role," *The New York Times,* March 21, 1996, A1–A22.

CHAPTER 5

1. Loevenhart, A. S., Lorenz, W. F., Martin, H. G., and Malone, J. Y., "Stimulation of Respiration by Sodium Cyanid [*sic*] and Its Clinical Application," *Archives of Internal Medicine*, 92 (1918), 109–129.
2. Furchgott, R. F., and Zawadzki, J. V., "The Obligatory Role of Endothelial Cells in the Relaxation of Arterial Smooth Muscle by Acetylcholine," *Nature*, 288 (1990), 373–376.
3. Moncada, S., Palmer, R. M. J., and Higgs, E. A., "The Discovery of Nitric Oxide as the Endogenous Nitrovasodilator," *Hypertension*, 12 (1988), 365–372.
4. Moncada, S., and Higgs, E. A., eds., *Nitric Oxide from L-Arginine: A Bioregulatory System* (Amsterdam: Elsevier Science Publishers, 1990).
5. Kolata, G., "Key Signal of Cells Found to Be a Common Gas," *The New York Times*, July 2, 1991, C1 and C6.
6. Rooke, T. W., and Hirsh, A. T., "Peripheral Vascular Disease." In Willerson, J. T., and Cohn, J. N., eds., *Cardiovascular Medicine* (New York: Churchill Livingstone, 1995), pp. 1162–1181. Figure 7.62, p. 1169.

CHAPTER 6

1. Hishikawa, K., Nakaki, T., Tsuda, M., Esumi, H., Ohshima, H., Suzuki, H., Saruta, T., and Kato, R., "Effect of Systemic L-arginine Administration on Hemodynamics and Nitric Oxide Release in Man," *Japan Heart Journal*, 33 (1992), 41–48.
2. Vallance, P., Patton, S., Bhagat, K., MacAllister, R., Radomski, M., Moncada, S., and Malinski, T., "Direct Measurement of Nitric Oxide in Human Beings," *The Lancet*, 346 (1995), 153–154.
3. Bacchus, R. A., and London, D. R., "The Measurement of Arginine in Plasma," *Clinica Chimica Acta*, 33 (1971), 479–482.
4. Kharitonov, S. A., Lubec, G., Hjelm, M., and Barnes, P. J., "L-Arginine Increases Exhaled Nitric Oxide in Normal Human Beings," *Clinical Sciences*, 88 (1995), 135–139.
5. Wennmalam, A., Benthin, G., Edlund, A., Jungersten, L., Kieler-Jensen, N., Lundin, S., Nathorst, U., Peterson, A.-S., and Waagstein, F., "Metabolism and Excretion of Nitric Oxide in Humans," *Circulation Research*, 73 (1993), 1121–1127.
6. Pennington, J. A. T., *Food Values* (New York: Harper Perennial, 1989).
7. Sodeman, W. A., and Sodeman, T. M., *Pathological Physiology*, 6th ed. (Philadelphia: W. B. Saunders, 1979).

CHAPTER 7

1. Kannel, W. B., Castelli, W. P., and McNamara, P. M., "Detection of the Coronary-Prone Adult: The Framingham Study," *Journal of the Iowa Medical Society,* 56 (1966), 26–34.
2. Cardillo, C., Kilcoyne, C. M., Cannon, R. O. III, and Panza, J. A., "Racial Differences in Nitric Oxide–Mediated Vasodilator Response to Mental Stress in the Forearm Circulation," *Hypertension,* 31 (1998), 1235–1239.
3. Hishikawa, K., Nakaki, T., Suzuki, H., Kato, R., and Saruta, T., "L-Arginine as an Antihypertensive Agent," *Journal of Cardiovascular Pharmacology,* Supplement 12, 20 (1992), S196–S197.
4. Nakaki, T., Hishikawa, K., Suzuki, H., Saruta, T., and Kato, R., "L-Arginine-Induced Hypotension," *The Lancet,* 336 (1990), 696.
5. Pagnotta, P., Germano, G., Filippo, G. G., Rosano, G. M. C., and Chierchia, S. L., "Oral L-Arginine Supplementation Improves Essential Arterial Hypertension," *Circulation* Supplement I, 96 (1997), 3014.
6. Rosano, G. M. C., Panina, G., Cerquetani, E., Leonardo, F., Pelliccia, F., Bonfigli, B., and Chierchia, S. L., "L-Arginine Improves Endothelial Function in Newly Diagnosed Hypertensives," *Journal of the American College of Cardiology* (Supplement A), 31 (1998), 262A.
7. Joint National Committee, "The 1988 Report of the Joint National Committee on Detection, Evaluation, and Treatment of High Blood Pressure," *Archives of Internal Medicine,* 148 (1988), 1023–1038.
8. Oliver, M. F., "Risks of Correcting the Risks of Coronary Disease and Stroke with Drugs," *The New England Journal of Medicine,* 306 (1982), 297–298.
9. Medical Research Council Working Party on Mild to Moderate Hypertension, W. S. Peart, chair, "Adverse Reactions to Bendrofluazide and Propranolol for the Treatment of Mild Hypertension," *The Lancet,* 2 (1981), 540–543.
10. Tomohiro, A., Kimura, S., He, H., Fujisawa, Y., Nishiyama, A., Kiyomoto, K., Aki, Y., Tamaki, T., and Abe, Y., "Regional Blood Flow in Dahl-Iwai Salt-Sensitive Rats and the Effects of L-Arginine Supplementation," *American Journal of Physiology,* 272 (1997), R1013–R1019.
11. Salazar, F. J., Alberola, A., Pinilla, J. M., Romero, J. C. and Quesada, T., "Salt-Induced Increase in Arterial Pressure during Nitric Oxide Synthesis Inhibition," *Hypertension,* 22 (1993), 49–55.
12. Brown, M. D., Dengel, D. R., and Supiano, M. A., "Nitric Oxide Biomarkers Are Associated with the Blood Pressure Lowering Effects of Dietary Sodium Restriction in Older Hypertensives," *Circulation* (Abstract I), 96 (1997), I-539.

CHAPTER 8

1. Gordon, T., and Kannel, W. B., "The Framingham, Massachusetts, Study Twenty Years Later." In Kessler, I. I., and Levin, M. L., eds., *The Community as an Epidemiologic Laboratory: A Casebook of Community Studies* (Baltimore: The Johns Hopkins University Press, 1970).

2. Boger, R. H., Bode-Boger, S. M., Brandes, R. P., Phivthong-ngam, L., Bohme, M., Nafe, R., Mugge, A., and Frolich, J. C., "Dietary L-Arginine Reduces the Progression of Atherosclerosis in Cholesterol Fed Rabbits: Comparison with Lovastatin," *Circulation*, 96 (1997), 1282–1290.

3. Newman, T. B., and Hulley, S. B., "Carcinogenicity of Lipid-Lowering Drugs," *Journal of the American Medical Association*, 275 (1996), 55–69.

4. Korbut, R., Bieron, K., and Gryglewski, R. J., "Effect of L-Arginine on Plasminogen-Activator Inhibitor in Hypertensive Patients with Hypercholesterolemia," *The New England Journal of Medicine*, 328 (1993), 287–288.

5. Stroes, E. S. G., Koomans, H. A., de Bruin, T. W. A., and Rabelink, T. J., "Vascular Function in the Forearm of Hypercholesterolaemic Patients off and on Lipid-Lowering Medication," *The Lancet*, 346 (1995), 467–471.

6. Hurson, M., Regan, M. C., Kirk, S. J., Wasserkrug, H. L., and A. Barbul, "Metabolic Effects of Arginine in a Healthy Elderly Population," *Journal of Parenteral & Enteral Nutrition*, 19 (1995), 227–230.

7. Esterbauer, H., Dieber-Rotheneder, M., Striegl, G., and Waeg, G., "Role of Vitamin E in Preventing Oxidation of Low-Density Lipoproteins," *American Journal of Clinical Nutrition*, 53 (Supplement) (1991), 314S–321S.

8. Hogg, N., Struck, A., Goss, S. P. A., Santanam, N., Joseph, J., Parthasarathy, S., and Kalyanaraman, B., "Inhibition of Macrophage-Dependent Low Density," *Journal of Lipid Research*, 36 (1993), 1756–1762.

9. Cooke, J. P., Singer, A. H., Tsao, P., Zera, P., Rowan, R. A., and Billingham, M. B., "Antiatherogenic Effects of L-Arginine in the Hypercholesterolemic Rabbit," *Journal of Clinical Investigation*, 90 (1992), 1168–1172.

10. Kuo, L., Davis, M. J., Cannon, M. S., and Chilian, W. M., "Pathophysiological Consequences of Atherosclerosis Extended into the Coronary Microcirculation: Restoration of Endothelium-Dependent Response by L-Arginine," *Circulation Research* 70 (1992), 465–476.

11. Bokelman, T. A., Wallhaus, T. R., White, T. E., Wolff, M. R., and Hanson, P., "Oral L-Arginine Augments Abnormal Endothelium-Dependent Skeletal Muscle Vasodilation in Patients with Coronary Artery Disease," *Circulation* Supplement I, 92 (1995), I–20.

12. Clarkson, P., Adams, M. R., Powe, A. J., Donald, A. E., McCredie, R.,

Robinson, J., Betteridge, D. J., Keech, A., Celermajer, D. S., and Dean-field, J. E., "Oral L-Arginine Improves Endothelium-Dependent Dilation in Hypercholesterolemic Young Adults," *Circulation,* Supplement I, 92 (1995), I–366.

13. Wolf, A., Zalpour, C., Theilmeier, G., Wang, B-Y., Ma, A., Anderson, B., Tsao, P. S., and Cooke, J. P., "Dietary L-Arginine Supplementation Normalizes Platelet Aggregation in Hypercholesterolemic Humans," *Journal of the American College of Cardiology,* 29 (1997), 479–485.

14. Zeiher, A. M., Schachinger, V., and Minners, J., "Long-Term Cigarette Smoking Impairs Endothelium-Dependent Coronary Arterial Vasodilator Function," *Circulation,* 92 (1995), 1094–1100.

15. Heitzer, T., Just, H., and Munzel, T., "Antioxidant Vitamin C Improves Endothelial Dysfunction in Chronic Smokers," *Circulation,* 94 (1996), 6–9.

CHAPTER 9

1. Hammond, I. W., Devereux, R. B., Alderman, M. H., et al., "The Prevalence and Correlates of Echocardiographic Left Ventricular Hypertrophy among Employed Patients with Uncomplicated Hypertension," *Journal of the American College of Cardiology,* 7 (1986), 639–650.

2. Frohlich, E. D., Apstein, C., Chobanian, A. V., Devereux, R. B., Dustan, H. P., Dzau, V., Fauad-Tarazi, F., Horan, M. J., Marcus, M., Massie, B., Pfeffer, M. A., Re, R. N., Roccella, E. J., Savage, D., and Shub, C., "The Heart in Hypertension," *The New England Journal of Medicine,* 327 (1992), 998–1008.

3. Rector, T. S., Bank, A. J., Mullen, K. A., Tchumperlin, L. K., Sih, R., Pillai, K., and Kubo, S. H., "Randomized, Double-Blind, Placebo-Controlled Study of Supplemental Oral L-Arginine in Patients with Heart Failure," *Circulation,* 93 (1996), 2135–2141.

4. Werns, S. W., Walton, J. A., Hsia, H. H., Nabel, E. G., Sanz, M. L., and Pitt, A., "Evidence of Endothelial Dysfunction in Angiographically Normal Coronary Arteries of Patients with Coronary Artery Disease," *Circulation,* 79 (1989), 287–291.

5. Alexander, R. W., "Hypertension and the Pathogenesis of Atherosclerosis," *Hypertension,* 25 (1995), 155–161.

6. Xu, C., Glagov, S., Zatina, M. A., and Zarins, C. K., "Hypertension Sustains Plaque Progression Despite Reduction of Hypercholesterolemia," *Hypertension,* 18 (1991), 123–129.

7. Pezza, V., Bernardini, F., Pezza, B., and Curione, M., "Study of Supplemental Oral L-Arginine (SOA) in Hypertensive Treated with Enalapril

(E) + Hydrochlorithiazide (H)," *American Journal of Hypertension* (Abstracts), 10 (1997), 179A.

CHAPTER 10

1. Mugge, A., Elwell, J. H., Peterson, T. E., Hofmeyer, T. G., Heistad, D. D., and Harrison, D. G., "Chronic Treatment with Polyethylene-Glycolate Superoxide Dismutase Partially Restores Endothelium-Dependent Vascular Relaxation in Cholesterol-Fed Rabbits," *Circulation Research*, 69 (1991), 1293–1300.

2. Blakeslee, S., "Surprise Discovery in Blood: Hemoglobin Has Bigger Role," *The New York Times*, March 21, 1996, A1–A22.

3. Stamler, J. S., Jia, L., Eu, J. P., McMahon, T. J., Demchenko, I. T., Bonaventura, J., Gerbert, K., and Piantadosi, C. A., "Blood Flow Regulation by S-Nitrosohemoglobin in the Physiological Oxygen Gradient," *Science*, 276 (1997), 2034–2036.

4. Ridker, P. M., Cushman, M., Stampfer, M. J., Tracy, R. P., and Hennekens, C. H., "Inflammation, Aspirin, and the Risk of Cardiovascular Disease in Apparently Healthy Men," *The New England Journal of Medicine*, 336 (1997), 973–979.

5. Kaplan, R. M., Sallis, J. F., and Patterson, T. L., *Health and Human Behavior* (New York: McGraw Hill, 1993).

6. Kelly, J. P., Kaufman, D. W., Jurgeon, J. M., Sheehan, J., Koff, R. S., and Shapiro, S., "Risk of Aspirin-Associated Major Upper Gastrointestinal Bleeding with Enteric Coated or Buffered Product," *The Lancet*, 348 (1996), 1413–1416.

7. Tuomainen, T.-P., Salonen, R., Nyyssonen, K., and Salonen, J., "Cohort Study of Relation Between Donating Blood and Risk of Myocardial Infarction in 2,682 Men in Eastern Finland," *British Medical Journal*, 314 (1997), 793–794.

8. Radomski, M. W., Palmer, R. M. J., and Moncada, S., "An L-Arginine/Nitric Oxide Pathway Present in Human Platelets Regulates Aggregation," *Proceedings of the National Academy of Sciences*, 87 (1990), 5193–5197.

9. Boder-Boger, S. M., Boger, R. H., Creutzig, A., Tsikas, D., Gutzki, F. M., Alexander, K., and Frolich, J. C., "L-Arginine Infusion Decreases Peripheral Arterial Resistance and Inhibits Platelet Aggregation in Healthy Subjects," *Clinical Science*, 87 (1994), 303–310.

10. Wolf, A., Zalpour, C., Theilmeier, G., Wang, B-Y., Ma, A., Anderson, B., Tsao, P. S., and Cooke, J. P., "Dietary L-Arginine Supplementation

Normalizes Platelet Aggregation in Hypercholesterolemic Humans," *Journal of the American College of Cardiology*, 29 (1997), 479–485.

CHAPTER 11

1. Talley, J. D., and Crawley, I. S., "Transdermal Nitrate, Penile Erection, and Spousal Headache," *Annals of Internal Medicine*, 103 (1985), 804.
2. Masters, William, and Johnson, Virginia, *Human Sexual Inadequacy* (Boston: Little Brown & Co., 1970).
3. Virag, R., Bouilly, P., and Frydman, D., "Is Impotence an Arterial Disorder?" *The Lancet*, 1 (1985), 181–184.
4. Rajfer, J., Aronson, W. J., Bush, P. A., Dorey, F. J., and Ignarro, L. J., "Nitric Oxide as a Mediator of Relaxation of the Corpus Cavernosum in Response to Nonadrenergic, Noncholinergic Neurotransmission," *The New England Journal of Medicine*, 326 (1992), 90–94.
5. Koshland, D. E., "The Molecule of the Year," *Science*, 258 (1992), 1861–1863.
6. Burnett, A. L., "Nitric Oxide in the Penis: Physiology and Pathology," *The Journal of Urology*, 157 (1997), 320–324.
7. Zorgniotti, A. W., and Lizza, E. F., "Effect of Large Doses of Nitric Oxide Precursor, L-Arginine, on Erectile Dysfunction," *International Journal of Impotence Research*, 6 (1994), 33–36.
8. Clarkson, P., Adams, M. R., Powe, A. J., Donald, A. E., McCredie, R., Robinson, J., McCarthy, S. N., Keech, A., Celermajer, D. S., and Deanfield, J. E., "Oral L-Arginine Improves Endothelium-Dependent Dilation in Hypercholesterolemic Young Adults," *Journal of Clinical Investigation*, 97 (1996), 1989–1994.
9. Gomaa, A., Shalaby, M., Osman, M., Eissa, M., Eizat, A., Mahmoud, M., and Mikhail, N., "Topical Treatment of Erectile Dysfunction: Randomized Double-Blind Placebo-Controlled Trial of Cream Containing Aminophylline, Isosorbide, and Co-Dergonic Mesulate," *British Medical Journal*, 312 (1996), 1512–1515.
10. "Much Ado About NO," *Harvard Health Letter*, Vol. 18 (1993), 6–7.
11. Blakeslee, S., "Chemical a Factor in Male Impotence," *The New York Times*, January 9, 1992, B10.
12. Adams, M. R., Jessup, W., and Celemajer, D. S., "Cigarette Smoking Is Associated with Increased Monocyte Adhesion to Endothelial Cells: Reversibility with Oral-L-Arginine but Not Vitamin C," *Journal of the American College of Cardiology*, 29 (1997), 491–496.

CHAPTER 12

1. Stuehr, D. J., and Marletta, M. A., "Mammalian Nitrate Biosynthesis: Mouse Macrophages Produce Nitrite and Nitrate in Response to *Escherichia Coli* Lipopolysaccharide," *Proceedings of the National Academy of Sciences*, 82 (1985), 7738–7742.

2. Park, K. G. M., Hayes, P. D., Garlick, P. J., Sewell, H., and Eremin, O., "Stimulation of Lymphocyte Natural Cytotoxicity by L-Arginine," *The Lancet*, 337 (1991), 645–646.

3. Green, S. J., and Nacy, C. A., "Antimicrobial and Immunopathologic Effects of Cytokine-Induced Nitric Oxide Synthesis," *Current Opinion in Infectious Diseases*, 6 (1993), 384–396.

4. De Groote, M. A., Granger, D., Xu, Y., Campbell, G., and Prince, R., "Genetic and Redox Determinants of Nitric Oxide Cytotoxicity in a *Salmonella typhimurium* Model," *Proceedings of the National Academy of Sciences (USA)*, 92 (1995), 6399–6403.

5. Dermer, G. B., *The Immortal Cell* (New York: Avery Publishing Group, 1994).

6. Takeda, Y., Tominaga, T., Tei, N., Kitamura, M., Taga, S., Murase, J., Taguchi, T., and Kiwatani, T., "Inhibitory Effect of L-Arginine on Growth of Rat Mammary Tumors Induced by 7,12-Dymethylbenz(a)anthracene," *Cancer Research*, 35 (1975), 2390–2393.

7. Fehleisen, V., "Ueber die Zuchtung der Erysipelkokken auf Kunstichen Narrborden und Ihre Uebertragbarkeit auf den Menschen," *Deutsche Medicinische Wochenschrift*, 8 (1882), 553–554.

8. Feinman, R., Henriksen-DeStephano, D., Tsujimoto, M., and J. Vilcek, "Tumor Necrosis Factor Is an Important Mediator of Tumor Cell Killing by Human Monocytes," *The Journal of Immunology*, 138 (1987), 635–640.

9. Drapier, J. C., Wietzerbin, J., and Hibbs, J. B., "Interferon-γ and Tumor Necrosis Factor Induce the L-Arginine-Dependent Cytotoxic Effector Mechanism in Murine Macrophages," *European Journal of Immunology*, 18 (1988), 1587–1592.

10. Hibbs, J. B., Vavrin, Z., and Taintor, R. R., "L-Arginine Is Required for Expression of the Activated Macrophage Effector Mechanism Causing Selective Metabolic Inhibition in Target Cells," *The Journal of Immunology*, 138 (1987), 550–565.

11. Kwon, N. S., Stuehr, D. J., and Nathan, C. F., "Inhibition of Tumor Cell Ribonucleotide Reductase by Macrophage-Derived Nitric Oxide," *Journal of Experimental Medicine*, 174 (1991), 761–767.

12. Albina, J. E., Mills, C. D., Barbul, A., Thirkill, C. E., Henry, W. L.,

Mastrofrancesco, B., and Caldwell, M. D., "Arginine Metabolism in Wounds," *American Journal of Physiology*, 254 (1988), E459–E467.

13. Barbul, A., Fishel, R. S., Shimazu, S., Wasserkrug, H. L., Yoshimura, N. N., Tao, R. C., and Efron, G., "Intravenous Alimentation with High Arginine Levels Improves Wound Healing and Immune Function," *Journal of Surgical Research*, 38 (1985), 228–334.

14. Albina, J. E., Mills, C. D., Barbul, A., Thirkill, C. E., Henry, W. L., Mastrofrancesco, B., and Caldwell, M. D., "Arginine Metabolism in Wounds," *American Journal of Physiology*, 254 (1988), E459–E467.

15. Barbul, A., Fishel, R. S., Shimazu, S., Wasserkrug, H. L., Yoshimura, N. N., Tao, R. C., and Efron, G., "Intravenous Alimentation with High Arginine Levels Improves Wound Healing and Immune Function," *Journal of Surgical Research*, 38 (1985), 228–334.

CHAPTER 13

1. Blakeslee, S., "Surprise Discovery in Blood: Hemoglobin Has Bigger Role," *The New York Times*, March 21, 1996, A1–A22.

2. Johnstone, M. T., Creager, S. J., Scales, K. M., Cusco, J. A., Lee, B. K., and Creager, M. A., "Impaired Endothelium-Dependent Vasodilation in Patients with Insulin-Dependent Diabetes Mellitus," *Circulation*, 88 (1993), 2510–2516.

3. Lubec, B., Hayn, M., Kitzmuller, E., Vierhapper, H., and Lubec, G., "L-Arginine Reduces Lipid Peroxidation in Patients with Diabetes Mellitus," *Free Radical Biology & Medicine*, 22 (1997), 355–357.

4. Joffe, I. I., Travers, K. E., Perreault, C. L., Hampton, T. G., Katz, S. E., Morgan, J. P., and Douglas, P. S., "Impaired Nitric Oxide Availability Contributes to the Cardiac Dysfunction of Diabetes," *Circulation* (abstracts), 96 (1997), I518.

5. Schmidt, H. H. H. W., Warner, T. D., Ishii, K., Sheng, H., and Murad, F., "Insulin Secretion from Pancreatic B Cells Caused by L-Arginine-Derived Nitrogen Oxides," *Science*, 255 (1992), 721–723.

6. Pieper, G. M., and Peltier, A., "Amelioration by L-Arginine of a Dysfunctional Arginine/Nitric Oxide Pathway in Diabetic Endothelium," *Journal of Cardiovascular Pharmacology*, 25 (1995), 397–403.

7. Buchanan, J. E., and Phillis, J. W., "The Role of Nitric Oxide in the Regulation of Cerebral Blood Flow," *Brain Research*, 610 (1993), 248–255.

8. Iadecola, C., "Regulation of the Cerebral Microcirculation during Neural Activity: Is Nitric Oxide the Missing Link?" *Trends in Neurosciences*, 16 (1993), 206–214.

9. Schuman, E. M., and Madison, D. V., "A Requirement for the Intercellular Messenger Nitric Oxide in Long-Term Potentiation," *Science*, 254 (1991), 1503–1506.

10. Thomas, T., Thomas, G., McLendon, C., Sutton, T., and Mullan, M., "β-Amyloid-Mediated Vasoactivity and Vascular Endothelial Damage," *Nature*, 380 (1996), 168–171.

11. Kuiper, M. A., Visser, J. J., Bergmans, P. L. M., Scheltens, P., and Wolters, E. C., "Decreased Cerebrospinal Fluid Nitrate Levels in Parkinson's Disease, Alzheimer's Disease and Multiple System Atrophy Patients," *Journal of Neurological Sciences*, 121 (1994), 46–49.

12. Rudman, D., Feller, A. G., Nagraj, H. S., Gergans, G. A., Lalitha, P. Y., Goldberg, A., Schlenker, R. A., Cohn, L., Rudman, I. W., and Mattson, D. E., "Effects of Human Growth Hormone in Men over 60 Years Old," *The New England Journal of Medicine*, 323 (1990), 1–6.

13. Merimee, T. J., Lillicrap, D. A., and Rabinowitz, D., "Effect of Arginine on Serum Levels of Human Growth-Hormone," *The Lancet*, 2 (1965), 668–670.

14. Braverman, E. R., and Pfeiffer, C. C., *The Healing Nutrients Within* (New Canaan, Conn.: Keats Publishing, Inc., 1987).

15. Copinschi, G., Wegienka, L. C., Hane, S., and Forsham, P. H., "Effect of Arginine on Serum Levels of Insulin and Growth Hormone in Obese Subjects," *Metabolism*, 16 (1967), 485–491.

16. Gordon, L., "L-Arginine May Help Reverse Age-Related Blood Vessel Damage," *The Medical Tribune*, 36 (1995), 4.

17. McCarthy, A. L., Woolfson, R. G., Raju, S. K., and Poston, L., "Abnormal Endothelial Cell Function of Resistance Arteries from Women with Preeclampsia," *American Journal of Obstetrics and Gynecology*, 168 (1993), 1323–1330.

18. Myatt, L., Brewer, A., and Brockman, D. E., "The Action of Nitric Oxide in the Perfused Human Fetal-Placental Circulation," *American Journal of Obstetrics and Gynecology*, 164 (1991), 687–692.

19. Izumi, H., Yallampalli, C., and Garfield, R. E., "Gestational Changes in L-Arginine-Induced Relaxation of Pregnant Rat and Human Myometrial Smooth Muscle," *American Journal of Obstetrics and Gynecology*, 169 (1993), 1327–1337.

20. de Belder, A., Lees, C., Martin, J., Moncada, S., and Campbell, S., "Treatment of HELLP Syndrome with Nitric Oxide Donor," *The Lancet*, 345 (1995), 124–125.

21. Izumi, H., Yallampalli, C., and Garfield, R. E., "Gestational Changes in

L-Arginine-Induced Relaxation of Pregnant Rat and Human Myometrial Smooth Muscle," *American Journal of Obstetrics and Gynecology*, 169 (1993), 1327–1337.

22. Kharitonov, S. A., Robbins, R. A., Yates, D., Keatings, V., and Barnes, P., "Acute and Chronic Effects of Cigarette Smoking on Exhaled Nitric Oxide," *American Journal of Respiratory and Critical Care Medicine*, 152 (1995), 602–612.

23. Gerlach, H., Pappert, D., Lewandowski, K., Rossaint, R., and Falke, K. J., "Long-Term Inhalation with Evaluated Low Doses of Nitric Oxide for Selective Improvement of Oxygenation in Patients with Adult Respiratory Distress Syndrome," *Intensive Care Medicine*, 19 (1993), 443–449.

24. O'Kelly, T., Brading, A., and Mortensen, N., "Nerve Mediated Relaxation of the Human Internal Anal Sphincter: The Role of Nitric Oxide," *Gut*, 34 (1993), 689–693.

25. Gorfine, S. R., "Treatment of Benign Anal Disease with Topical Nitroglycerin," *Diseases of the Colon & Rectum*, 38 (1995), 453–457.

26. Gorfine, S. R., "Topical Nitroglycerin Therapy for Anal Fissures and Ulcers," *The New England Journal of Medicine*, 333 (1995), 1156–1157.

27. Lund, J. N., and Scholefield, J. H., "A Randomised, Prospective, Double-Blind Placebo-Controlled Trial of Glyceryl Trinitrate Ointment in Treatment of Anal Fissure," *The Lancet*, 349 (1997), 11–14.

28. Watson, S. J., Kamm, M. A., Nicholls, R. J., and Phillips, R. K. S., "Topical Glyceryl Trinitrate in the Treatment of Chronic Anal Fissure," *British Journal of Surgery*, 83 (1996), 771–775.

29. Leary, W. E., "Finding Intrigues Sickle Cell Experts," *The New York Times*, April 23, 1996, C5.

CHAPTER 14

1. Hanington, E., "The Platelet Theory," in J. N. Blau, (ed.), *Migraine* (Baltimore: The Johns Hopkins University Press, 1987), 265–302.

2. Lassen, L. H., Shina, M., Christiansen, I., Ulrich, V., and Olesen, J., "Nitric Oxide Inhibition in Migraine," *The Lancet*, 349 (1997), 401–402.

3. Finkel, M. S., Laghrissi-Thode, F., Pollock, B. G., and Rong, J., "Paroxetine Is a Novel Nitric Oxide Synthase Inhibitor," *Psychopharmacology Bulletin*, 32 (1996), 653–658.

4. Winsor, T., and Beckett, J. C., "Biological Effects of Ionized Air in Man," *American Journal of Physical Medicine*, 37 (1958), 83–89.

5. Giannini, A. J., Castellani, S., and Dvoredsky, A. E., "Anxiety States: Re-

lationship to Athmospheric Cations and Serotonin," *Journal of Clinical Psychiatry,* 44 (1983), 262–264.

6. Boughton-Smith, N. K., Evans, S. M., Hawkey, C. J., Cole, A. T., Balsitis, M., Whittle, B. J. R., and Moncada, S., "Nitric Oxide Synthase Activity in Ulcerative Colitis and Crohn's Disease," *The Lancet,* 342 (1993), 338–340.

7. Lundberg, J. O. N., Hellstrom, P. M., Lundberg, J. M., and Alving, K., "Greatly Increased Luminal Nitric Oxide in Ulcerative Colitis," *The Lancet,* 344 (1994), 1673–1674.

8. Hogaboam, C. M., Jacobson, K., Collins, S. M., and Blennerhassett, M. G., "The Selective Beneficial Effects of Nitric Oxide Inhibition in Experimental Colitis," *American Journal of Physiology,* 268 (1995), G673–G684.

9. Kaur, H., and Halliwell, B., "Evidence for Nitric Oxide-Mediated Oxidative Damage in Chronic Inflammation. Nitrotyrosine in Serum and Synovial Fluid from Rheumatoid Patients," *Federation of European Biochemical Societies,* 350 (1994), 9–12.

10. Merrill, J. E., Ignarro, L. J., Sherman, M. P., Melinek, J., and Lane, T. E., "Microglial Cell Cytotoxicity of Oligodendrocytes Is Mediated through Nitric Oxide," *Journal of Immunology,* 151 (1993), 2132–2141.

11. Giovannoni, G., Heales, S. J. R., Silver, N. C., O'Riordan, J., Miller, R. F., Land, J. M., Clark, J. B., and Thompson, E. J., "Raised Serum Nitrate and Nitrite Levels in Patients with Multiple Sclerosis," *Journal of Neurological Sciences,* 145 (1997), 77–81.

12. Cho-Chung, Y. S., Clair, T., Bodwin, J. S., and Berghoffer, B., "Growth Arrest and Morphological Change in Human Breast Cancer Cells by Dibutyryl Cyclic AMP and L-Arginine," *Science,* 214 (1981), 77–79.

13. Cho-Chung, Y. S., Clair, T., Bodwin, J. S., and Hill, D. M., "Arrest of Mammary Tumor Growth in Vivo by L-Arginine: Stimulation of NAD-Dependent Activation of Adenylate Cyclase," *Biochemical and Biophysical Research Communication,* 95 (1980), 1306–1313.

14. Cho-Chung, Y. S., Clair, T., Bodwin, J. S., and Hill, D. M., "Arrest of Mammary Tumor Growth in Vivo by L-Arginine: Stimulation of NAD-Dependent Activation of Adenylate Cyclase," *Biochemical and Biophysical Research Communication,* 95 (1980), 1306–1313.

15. Brittenden, J., Park, K. G. M., Heys, S. D., Ashby, C. R. J., Ah-See, A. K., and Eremin, O., "L-Arginine Stimulates Host Defense in Patients with Breast Cancer," *Surgery,* 115 (1994), 205–212.

16. Matsumoto, A., Ogura, K., Hirata, Y., Kakoki, M., Watanabe, F., Takenata, K., Shiratori, Y., Momomura, S.-I., and Omata, M., "Increased Nitric Oxide in the Exhaled Air of Patients with Decompensated Liver Cirrhosis," *Annals of Internal Medicine,* 123 (1995), 110–113.

17. Rolla, G., Brussino, L., Colagrande, P., Scappaticci, E., Morello, M., Bergerone, S., Ottobrelli, A., Cerutti, E., Polizzi, S., and Bucca, C., "Exhaled Nitric Oxide and Impaired Oxygenation in Cirrhotic Patients before and after Liver Transplantation," *Annals of Internal Medicine,* 129 (1998), 375–378.

18. Martin, P.-Y., Gines, P., and Schrier, R. W., "Nitric Oxide as a Mediator of Hemodynamic Abnormalities and Sodium and Water Retention in Cirrhosis," *The New England Journal of Medicine,* 339 (1998), 533–541.

19. Cobb, J. P., and Danner, R. L., "Grand Rounds at the Clinical Center of the National Institutes of Health: Nitric Oxide and Septic Shock," *Journal of the American Medical Association,* 275 (1996), 1192–1196.

BIBLIOGRAPHY

Adams, M. R.; Forsyth, C. J.; Jessup, W.; Robinson, J.; and Celermajer, D. S. "Oral L-Arginine Inhibits Platelet Aggregation but Does Not Enhance Endothelium-Dependent Dilation in Healthy Young Men." *Journal of the American College of Cardiology,* 26 (1995) 1054–1061.

Adams, M. R.; Jessup, W.; and Celemajer, D. S. "Cigarette Smoking Is Associated with Increased Monocyte Adhesion to Endothelial Cells: Reversibility with Oral-L-Arginine but Not Vitamin C." *Journal of the American College of Cardiology,* 29 (1997) 491–496.

Adams, M. R.; Jessup, W.; McCredie, R.; Robinson, J.; Sullivan, D. S.; and Celermajer, D. S. "Oral L-Arginine Improves Endothelium-Dependent Dilatation and Reduces Monocyte Adhesion to Endothelial Cells in Young Men with Coronary Artery Disease." Supplement to the *Journal of the American College of Cardiology,* 29 (1997) 387A.

Adams, M. R.; McCredie, R.; Jessup, W.; Robinson, J.; Sullivan, D.; and Celermajer, D. S. "Oral L-Arginine Improves Endothelium-Dependent Dilation and Reduces Monocyte Adhesion to Endothelial Cells in Young Men with Coronary Artery Disease." *Atherosclerosis,* 129 (1997) 261–269.

Adamson, D. C.; Wildemann, B.; Sasaki, M.; Glass, J. D.; McArthur, J. C.; Christov, V. I.; Dawson, T. M.; and Dawson, V. L. "Immunologic NO Synthase: Elevation in Severe AIDS Dementia and Induction of HIV-1 gp41." *Science,* 274 (1996) 1917–1921.

Albina, J. E.; Caldwell, M. D.; Henry, W. L.; and Mills, C. D. "Regulation of Macrophage Function by L-Arginine." *Journal of Experimental Medicine,* 169 (1989) 1021–1029.

Albina, J. E.; Mills, C. D.; Barbul, A.; Thirkill, C. E.; Henry, W. L.; Mastrofrancesco, B.; and Caldwell, M. D. "Arginine Metabolism in Wounds." *American Journal of Physiology,* 254 (1988) E459–E467.

Alexander, R. W. "Hypertension and the Pathogenesis of Atherosclerosis." *Hypertension,* 25 (1995) 155–161.

Alving, K.; Weitzberg, E.; and Lundberg, J. M. "Increased Amounts of Nitric

Oxide in Exhaled Air of Asthmatics." *European Respiratory Journal*, 6 (1993) 1368–1370.

American Dietetics Association Handbook of Clinical Dietetics. New Haven: Yale University Press, 1981.

"Another Role for Nitric Oxide." *AIDS Weekly*, October 18, 1993, 12.

Anthony, M. "Amine Metabolism in Migraine." In Blau, J. N. (ed.) *Migraine*. Baltimore: The Johns Hopkins University Press, 1987, 265–302.

Bacchus, R. A., and London, D. R. "The Measurement of Arginine in Plasma." *Clinica Chimica Acta*, 33 (1971) 479–482.

Bailar, J. C., and Gornick, H. L. "Cancer Undefeated." *The New England Journal of Medicine*, 336 (1997) 1569–1574.

Baldweg, T.; Sooranna, S.; Das, I.; Catalan, J.; and Gazzard, B. "Serum Nitrite Concentration Suggests a Role for Nitric Oxide in AIDS," *AIDS*, 10 (1996) 451–452.

Barbul, A. "Arginine: Biochemistry and Therapeutic Implications." *Journal of Parenteral and Enteral Nutrition*, 10 (1986) 227–238.

Barbul, A.; Fishel, R. S.; Shimazu, S.; Wasserkrug, H. I.; Yoshimura, N. N.; Tao, R. C.; and Efron, G. "Intravenous Alimentation with High Arginine Levels Improves Wound Healing and Immune Function." *Journal of Surgical Research*, 38 (1985) 228–334.

Barbul, A.; Rettura, G.; Levenson, S. M.; and Seifert, E. "Arginine: A Thymotropic and Wound-Healing Promoting Agent." *Surgical Forum*, 28 (1977) 101–103.

Barbul, A.; Sisto, D. A.; Wasserkrug, H. L.; Yoshimura, N. N.; and Efron, G. "Metabolic and Immune Effects of Arginine in Postinjury Hyperalimentation." *The Journal of Trauma*, 21 (1981) 970–974.

Barbul, A.; Wasserkrug, H. L.; Yoshimura, N.; Tao, R.; and Efron, G. "High Arginine Levels in Intravenous Hyperalimentation Abrogate Post-Traumatic Immune Suppression." *Journal of Surgical Research*, 36 (1984) 620–624.

Barinaga, M. "Learning by Diffusion: Nitric Oxide May Spread Memories." *Nature*, 263 (1994) 466.

Barlet, A.; Albrecht, J.; Aubert, A.; Fischer, M.; Grof, F.; Grothuesmann, H. G.; Masson, J.; Mazeman, E.; Mermon, R.; Reichelt, H.; Schonmetzler, F.; and Suhler, A. "Wirksamkeit eines extraktes aus pygeum africanum in der medikamentosen therapie von miktionsstorungen infolge einer benignen prostatahyperplasie: Bewertung objektiver und subjektiver parameter." *Wiener Klinische Wochenschrift*, 102 (1990) 667–673.

Barnes, P. J., and Belvisi, M. G. "Nitric Oxide and Lung Disease." *Thorax*, 48 (1993) 1034–1043.

Bartram, T. *Encyclopedia of Herbal Medicine.* Christchurch, Dorset, Great Britain, 1995. This book includes mention of black cohosh, chamomile, garlic, hawthorn, nettles, and valerian.

Beckman, J. S. "The Double-Edged Role of Nitric Oxide in Brain Function and Superoxide-Mediated Injury." *Journal of Developmental Physiology,* 15 (1991) 53–59.

Belvisi, M. G.; Stretton, C. D.; Yacoub, M.; and Barnes, P. J. "Nitric Oxide Is the Endogenous Neurotransmitter of Bronchodilator Nerves in Humans." *European Journal of Pharmacology,* 210 (1992) 221–222.

Berkow, R. (ed.) *The Merck Manual,* 14th ed. Rahway, N.J.: Merck Sharp & Dohme Research Laboratories, 1982.

Berkowitz, G. S., and Papiernik, E. "Epidemiology of Preterm Birth." *Epidemiologic Reviews,* 15 (1993) 414–443.

Besset, A.; Bonardet, A.; Rondouin, G.; Descomps, B.; and Passouant, P. "Increase in Sleep-Related GH and Prl Secretion after Chronic Arginine Aspartate Administration in Man." *Acta Endocrinologica,* 99 (1982) 18–23.

Black, R. S.; Flint, S.; Lees, C.; and Campbell, S. "Preterm Labour and Delivery." *European Journal of Pediatrics,* 155 [Suppl. 2] (1996) S2–S7.

Blakeslee, S. "Chemical a Factor in Male Impotence." *The New York Times,* January 9, 1992, B10.

———. "Surprise Discovery in Blood: Hemoglobin Has Bigger Role." *The New York Times,* March 21, 1996, A1–A22.

———. "What Controls Blood Flow?" *The New York Times,* July 22, 1997, C1 and C8.

Bland, J. *Nutritional Improvement of Health Outcomes—The Inflammatory Disorders.* Gig Harbor, Wash.: HealthComm, Inc., 1997.

Bland, J. S. *New Perspectives in Nutritional Therapies.* Gig Harbor, Wash.: HealthComm, Inc., 1996.

Boder-Boger, S. M.; Boger, R. H.; Alfke, H.; Heinzel, D.; Tsikas, D.; Creutzig, A.; Alexander, K.; and Frolich, J. C. "L-Arginine Induces Nitric Oxide-Dependent Vasodilation in Patients with Critical Limb Ischemia: A Randomized, Controlled Study." *Circulation,* 93 (1996) 89–95.

Boder-Boger, S. M.; Boger, R. H.; Creutzig, A.; Tsikas, D.; Gutzki, F. M.; Alexander, K.; and Frolich, J. C. "L-Arginine Infusion Decreases Peripheral Arterial Resistance and Inhibits Platelet Aggregation in Healthy Subjects." *Clinical Science,* 87 (1994) 303–310.

Boger, R. H.; Boder-Boger, S. M.: Brandes, R. P.; Phivthong-ngam, L.; Bohme, M.; Nafe, R.; Mugge, A.; and Frolich, J. C. "Dietary L-Arginine Reduces the Progression of Atherosclerosis in Cholesterol Fed Rabbits: Comparison with Lovastatin." *Circulation,* 96 (1997) 1282–1290.

Bokelman, T. A.; Walhaus, T. R.; White, T. E.; Wolff, M. R.; and Hanson, P. "Oral L-Arginine Augments Abnormal Endothelium-Dependent Skeletal Muscle Vasodilation in Patients with Coronary Artery Disease." *Circulation* (Supplement I), 92 (1995) I–19.

Bone, R. C. "A New Therapy for the Adult Respiratory Distress Syndrome." *The New England Journal of Medicine,* 328 (1993) 431–432.

Boughton-Smith, N. K.; Evans, S. M.; Hawkey, C. J.; Cole, A. T.; Balsitis, M.; Whittle, B. J. R.; and Moncada, S. "Nitric Oxide Synthase Activity in Ulcerative Colitis and Crohn's Disease." *The Lancet,* 342 (1993) 338–340.

Bower, R. H.; Cerra, F. B.; Bershadsky, B.; Licari, J. J.; Hoyt, D. B.; Jensen, G. L.; Van Buren, C. T.; Rothkopf, M. M.; and Adelsberg, B. R. "Early Enteral Administration of a Formula (Impact) Supplemented with Arginine, Nucleotides, and Fish Oil in Intensive Care Unit Patients: Result of a Multicenter, Prospective, Randomized, Clinical Trial." *Critical Care Medicine,* 23 (1995) 436–449.

Bradbury, J. "Antihypertensive Drugs Can Affect Intellectual Function." *The Lancet,* 350 (1997) 1753.

Braverman, E. R., and Pfeiffer, C. C. *The Healing Nutrients Within.* New Canaan, Conn.: Keats Publishing, Inc., 1987.

Brittenden, J.; Heys, S. D.; Miller, I.; Sakar, T. K.; Hutcheon, A. W.; Needham, G.; Gilbert, F.; McKean, M.; Ah-See, A. K.; and Eremin, O. "Dietary Supplementation with L-Arginine in Patients with Breast Cancer (> 4 cm) Receiving Multimodality Treatment: Report of a Feasibility Study." *British Journal of Cancer,* 69 (1994) 918–921.

Brittenden, J.; Park, K. G. M.; Heys, S. D.; Ashby, C. R. J.; Ah-See, A. K.; and Eremin, O. "L-Arginine Stimulates Host Defense in Patients with Breast Cancer." *Surgery,* 115 (1994) 205–212.

Brody, J. E. "Impotence: More Options, More Experts, More Success." *The New York Times,* August 9, 1995, C8.

Brown, M. D.; Dengel, D. R.; and Supiano, M. A. "Nitric Oxide Biomarkers Are Associated with the Blood Pressure Lowering Effects of Dietary Sodium Restriction in Older Hypertensives." *Circulation* (Abstract I), 96 (1997) I-539.

Brown, T. M., and Skop, B. P. "Nitroglycerin in the Treatment of Serotonin Syndrome" (letter). *Annals of Pharmacology,* 30 (1996) 191–192.

Brush, J. E., Jr.; Cannon, R. O., III; Schenke, W. H. et al. "Angina Due to Coronary Microvascular Disease in Hypertensive Patients without Left Ventricular Hypertrophy." *The New England Journal of Medicine,* 319 (1988) 1302–1307.

Buchanan, J. E., and Phillis, J. W. "The Role of Nitric Oxide in the Regulation of Cerebral Blood Flow." *Brain Research,* 610 (1993) 248–255.

Buhimschi, I.; Yallampalli, C.; Dong, Y.-L.; and Garfield, R. E. "Involvement of a Nitric Oxide-Cyclic Guanosine Monophosphate Pathway in Control of Human Uterine Contractility during Pregnancy." *American Journal of Obstetrics and Gynecology,* 172 (1995) 1577–1584.

Buja, M. L. "Basic Mechanisms of Atherosclerosis." In Willerson, J. T., and Cohn, J. N. (eds.). *Cardiovascular Medicine.* New York: Churchill Livingstone, 1995.

Bukrinsky, M. I.; Nottet, H. S. L. M.; Schmidtmayerova, H.; Dubrosky, L.; Flanagan, C. R.; Mullins, M. E.; Lipton, S. A.; and Gendelman, H. E. "Regulation of Nitric Oxide Synthase Activity in Human Immunodeficiency Virus Type 1 (HIV-1)-Infected Monocytes: Implications for HIV-Associated Neurological Disease." *Journal of Experimental Medicine,* 181 (1995) 735–745.

Burnett, A. L. "Nitric Oxide in the Penis: Physiology and Pathology." *The Journal of Urology,* 157 (1997) 320–324.

Burns, R. A.; and Milner, J. A. "Effect of Arginine on the Carcinogenicity of 7,12-Dimethylbenz[a]-Anthracene and N-Methyl-N-Nitrosourea." *Carcinogenesis,* 5 (1984) 1539–1542.

Bushinsky, D. A.; and Gennari, F. J. "Life-Threatening Hyperkalemia Induced by Arginine." *Annals of Internal Medicine,* 89 (1978) 632–634.

Calver, A.; Collier, J.; and Vallance, P. "Dilator Action of Arginine in Human Peripheral Vasculature." *Clinical Science,* 81 (1991) 695–700.

Cameron, I. T.; van Papendorp, C. L.; Palmer, R. M. J.; Smith, S. K.; and Moncada, S. "Relationship between Nitric Oxide Synthesis and Increase in Systolic Blood Pressure in Women with Hypertension in Pregnancy." *Hypertension in Pregnancy,* 12 (1993) 85–92.

Carani, C. "Urological and Sexual Evaluation of Treatment of Benign Prostatic Disease Using *Pygeum Africanum* at High Doses." *Archiva Italiano di Utologia, Nefrologia, Andrologia,* 63 (1991) 341–345.

Cardillo, C.; Kilcoyne, C. M.; Cannon, R. O., III; and Panza, J. A. "Racial Differences in Nitric Oxide-Mediated Vasodilator Response to Mental Stress in the Forearm Circulation." *Hypertension,* 31 (1998) 1235–1239.

Carroll, L. "Nitric Oxide Helps 'Blue Babies' Avoid Risky Operation." *Medical Tribune,* June 20, 1996, p. 16.

Casino, P. R.; Kilcoyne, C. M.; Quyyumi, A. A.; Hoeg, J. M.; and Panza, J. A. "Investigation of Decreased Availability of Nitric Oxide Precursor as a Mechanism Responsible for Impaired Endothelium-Dependent Vasodilation in Hypercholesterolemic Patients." *Journal of the American College of Cardiology,* 23 (1994) 844–850.

Celermajer, D. S.; Sorensen, K. E.; Georgakopoulos, D.; Bull, K.; Thomas, O.; Robinson, J.; and Deanfield, J. E. "Cigarette Smoking Is Associated with Dose-Related and Potentially Reversible Impairment of Endothelium-Dependent Dilation in Healthy Young Adults." *Circulation,* 88 (Part I) (1993) 2149–2155.

Champault, G.; Patel, J. C.; and Bonnard, A. M. "A Double-Blind Trial of an Extract of the Plant *Serenoa repens* in Benign Prostatic Hyperplasia." *British Journal of Pharmacology,* 18 (1984) 461–462.

Chauhan, A.; More, R. S.; Mullins, P. A.; Taylor, G.; Petch, M. C.; and Schofield, P. M. "Aging-Associated Endothelial Dysfunction in Humans Is Reversed by L-Arginine." *Circulation* (Supplement) 92 (1995) I-K.

Chen, P., and Sanders, P. W. "L-Arginine Abrogates Salt-Sensitive Hypertension in Dahl/Rapp Rats." *Journal of Clinical Investigation,* 88 (1991) 1559–1567.

Cho-Chung, Y. S.; Clair, T.; Bodwin, J. S.; and Berghoffer, B. "Growth Arrest and Morphological Change in Human Breast Cancer Cells by Dibutyryl Cyclic AMP and L-Arginine." *Science,* 214 (1981), 77–79.

Cho-Chung, Y. S.; Clair, T.; Bodwin, J. S.; and Hill, D. M. "Arrest of Mammary Tumor Growth in Vivo by L-Arginine: Stimulation of NAD-Dependent Activation of Adenylate Cyclase." *Biochemical and Biophysical Research Communication,* 95 (1980) 1306–1313.

Clarkson, P.; Adams, M. R.; Powe, A. J.; Donald, A. E.; McCredie, R.; Robinson, J.; McCarthy, S. N.; Keech, A.; Celermajer, D. S.; and Deanfield, J. E. "Oral L-Arginine Improves Endothelium-Dependent Dilation in Hypercholesterolemic Young Adults." *Journal of Clinical Investigation,* 97 (1996) 1989–1994.

Cobb, J. P., and Danner, R. L. "Grand Rounds at the Clinical Center of the National Institutes of Health: Nitric Oxide and Septic Shock." *Journal of the American Medical Association,* 275 (1996) 1192–1196.

Coiro, V.; Volpi, R.; Capretti, L.; Speroni, G.; Caffarri, G.; and Chiodera, P. "Involvement of Nitric Oxide in Arginine, but Not Glucose, Induced Insulin Secretion." *Clinical Endocrinology,* 46 (1997) 115–119.

Collaborative Group for the Study of Stroke in Young Women. "Oral Contraception and Increased Risk of Cerebral Ischemia or Thrombosis." *The New England Journal of Medicine,* 288 (1973) 871–878.

Cooke, J. P.; Singer, A. H.; Tsao, P.; Zera, P.; Rowan, R. A.; and Billingham, M. B. "Antiatherogenic Effects of L-Arginine in the Hypercholesterolemic Rabbit." *Journal of Clinical Investigation,* 90 (1992) 1168–1172.

Copinschi, G.; Wegienka, L. C.; Hane, S.; and Forsham, P. H. "Effect of Arginine on Serum Levels of Insulin and Growth Hormone in Obese Subjects." *Metabolism*, 16 (1967) 485–491.

Crawford, M. H., and Sorensen, S. G. "Noninvasive Techniques." In Stein, J. H. ed., *Internal Medicine*. Little, Brown and Co., 1983, pp. 449–460.

Creager, M. A.; Gallagher, S. J.; Girerd, X. J.; Coleman, S. M.; Dzau, V. J.; and Cooke, J. P. "L-Arginine Improves Endothelium-Dependent Vasodilation in Hypercholesterolemic Humans." *Journal of Clinical Investigation*, 90 (1992) 1248–1253.

Critselis, A.; Rettura, A.; Barbul, A.; and Seifert, E. "Arginine Inhibits a Viral Tumor." *Federation Proceedings*, 36 (Abstract 4711) (1977) 1163.

Culotta, E., and Koshland, Jr., D. E. "NO News Is Good News." *Science*, 258 (1992) 1862–1865.

Dalessio, D. J., ed. *Wolff's Headache and Other Head Pain*. New York: Oxford University Press, 1980.

Daly, J.; Reynolds, J.; Thom, A.; Kinsley, L.; Dietrick-Gallagher, M.; Shou, J.; and Ruggieri, B. "Immune and Metabolic Effects of Arginine in the Surgical Patient." *Annals of Surgery*, 208 (1988) 512–523.

Dawson, T. M., and Dawson, V. L. "Nitric Oxide: Actions and Pathological Roles." *The Neuroscientist*, 1 (1995) 7–18.

de Belder, A.; Lees, C.; Martin, J.; Moncada, S.; and Campbell, S. "Treatment of HELLP Syndrome with Nitric Oxide Donor." *The Lancet*, 345 (1995) 124–125.

De Groote, M. A.; Granger, D.; Xu, Y.; Campbell, G.; and Prince, R. "Genetic and Redox Determinants of Nitric Oxide Cytotoxicity in a *Salmonella typhimurium* Model." *Proceedings of the National Academy of Sciences (USA)*, 92 (1995) 6399–6403.

De Palma, R. G. "New Developments in the Diagnosis and Treatment of Impotence." *Western Journal of Medicine*, 164 (1996) 54.

Dermer, G. B. *The Immortal Cell*. New York: Avery Publishing Group, 1994.

Di Silvero, F.; D'Eramo, G.; Lubrano, C.; Flammia, G. P.; Sciarra, A.; Palma, E.; Caponera, M.; and Sciarra, F. "Evidence that Serenoa repens Extract Displays Antiestrogenic Activity in Prostatic Tissue of Benign Prostatic Hypertrophy Patients." *European Urology*, 21 (1992) 309–314.

Din-Yuan, A. T.; Higenbottam, T. W.; Pepke-Zaba, J.; Cremona, G.; Butt, A. Y.; Large, S. R.; Wells, F. C.; and Wallwork, J. "Impairment of Endothelium-Dependent Pulmonary-Artery Relaxation in Chronic Obstructive Lung Disease." *The New England Journal of Medicine*, 324 (1991) 1539–1547.

Donkervoort, T.; Sterling, A.; van Ness, J.; and Donker, P. J. "A Clinical and Urodynamic Study of Tadenan in Treatment of Benign Prostatic Hypertrophy." *European Urology*, 8 (1977) 218–225.

Dorgan, C. A. *Statistical Record of Health and Medicine.* New York: Thompson Publishing Co., 1995.

Drapier, J. C.; Wietzerbin, J.; and Hibbs, J. B. "Interferon-g and Tumor Necrosis Factor Induce the L-Arginine-Dependent Cytotoxic Effector Mechanism in Murine Macrophages." *European Journal of Immunology*, 18 (1988) 1587–1592.

Drexler, H.; Zeiher, A. M.; Meinzer, K.; and Just, H. "Correction of Endothelial Dysfunction in Coronary Microcirculation of Hypercholesterolaemic Patients by L-Arginine." *The Lancet*, 338 (1991) 1546–1550.

Dubovsky, S. "Nonserotonin Effect of an SSRI." *Journal Watch for Psychiatry*, 3 (1997) 23.

Egashira, K.; Hirooka, Y.; Kuga, T.; Mohri, M.; and Takeshita, A. "Effects of L-Arginine Supplementation on Endothelium-Dependent Coronary Vasodilation in Patients with Angina Pectoris and Normal Coronary Arteriograms." *Circulation*, 94 (1996) 130–134.

Egger, J.; Carter, C. M.; Soothill, J. F.; and Wilson, J. "Oligoantigenic Diet Treatment of Children with Epilepsy and Migraine." *Journal of Pediatrics*, 114 (1989) 51–58.

Epstein, R. H. "The New Miracle Drug May Be—Smog." *Business Week*, December 5, 1994, pp. 108–109.

Erslev, A. J., and Gabuzda, T. S. *Pathophysiology of Blood.* Philadelphia: W. B. Saunders, 1975.

Esterbauer, H.; Dieber-Rotheneder, M.; Striegl, G.; and Waeg, G. "Role of Vitamin E in Preventing Oxidation of Low-Density Lipoproteins." *American Journal of Clinical Nutrition*, 53 (Supplement) (1991) 314S–321S.

Fackelmann, K. "Cholesterol and Cancer." *Science News*, 149 (1996) 136–138.

———. "Gastrointestinal Blues: Research Finds Bugs that Inflame the Human Gut." *Science News*, 150 (1996) 302–303.

Faraci, F. M. "Regulation of Cerebral Circulation by Endothelium." *Pharmacology & Therapeutics*, 56 (1992) 1–22.

Faraci, F. M., and Brian, J. E., Jr. "Nitric Oxide in the Cerebral Circulation." *Stroke*, 25 (1994) 692–703.

Farmer, A. J., and Gotto, A. M. "Atherosclerosis: Pathogenesis and Risk Factors," fig. 7.36, p. 1104. In Willerson, J. T., and Cohen, J. N., eds., *Cardiovascular Medicine.* New York: Churchill Livingstone, 1995, pp. 1101–1113.

Fehleisen, V. "Ueber die Zuchtung der Erysipelkokken auf Kunstichen Narr-borden und Ihre Uebertragbarkeit auf den Menschen." *Deutsche Medicinische Wochenschrift*, 8 (1882) 553–554.

Feinman, R.; Henriksen-DeStephano, D.; Tsujimoto, M.; and Vilcek, J. "Tumor Necrosis Factor Is an Important Mediator of Tumor Cell Killing by Human Monocytes." *The Journal of Immunology*, 138 (1987) 635–640.

Finkel, M. S.; Laghrissi-Thode, F.; Pollock, B. G.; and Rong, J. "Paroxetine Is a Novel Nitric Oxide Synthase Inhibitor." *Psychopharmacology Bulletin*, 32 (1996) 653–658.

Finkelstein, J. W.; Roffwarg, H. P.; Boyar, R. M.; Kream, J.; and Hellman, L. "Age-Related Change in the Twenty-Four-Hour Spontaneous Secretion of Growth Hormone." *Journal of Endocrinology and Metabolism*, 35 (1972) 665–670.

Flavahan, N. N. "Atherosclerosis or Lipoprotein-Induced Endothelial Dysfunction: Potential Mechanism Underlying Reduction in EDRF/Nitric Oxide Activity." *Circulation*, 85 (1992) 927–1938.

Franklin, M.; Krauthamer, M.; Tai, A. R.; and Pinchot, A. *The Heart Doctors' Heart Book*. New York: Grossett and Dunlap, 1974.

Fried, R. *The Psychology and Physiology of Breathing in Behavioral Medicine, Clinical Psychology and Psychiatry*. New York: Plenum Press, 1993.

Fried, R., and Carlton, R. M. "Intracellular Magnesium Deficiency in Idiopathic Epilepsy." *Journal of the American College of Nutrition* (abstract), 4 (1984) 429–430.

Frohlich, E. D.; Apstein, C.; Chobanian, A. V.; Devereux, R. B.; Dustan, H. P.; Dzau, V.; Fauad-Tarazi, F.; Horan, M. J.; Marcus, M.; Massie, B.; Pfeffer, M. A.; Re, R. N.; Roccella, E. J.; Savage, D.; and Shub, C. "The Heart in Hypertension." *The New England Journal of Medicine*, 327 (1992) 998–1008.

Frostell, C.; Fratacci, M.-D.; Wain, J. C.; Jones, R.; and Zapol, W. M. "Inhaled Nitric Oxide: A Selective Pulmonary Vasodilator Reversing Hypoxic Pulmonary Vasoconstriction." *Circulation*, 83 (1991) 2038–2047.

Furberg, C. D.; Byington, R. P.; and Riley, W. "B-Mode Ultrasound: A Noninvasive Method for Assessing Atherosclerosis." In Willerson, J. T., and Cohn, J. N., eds., *Cardiovascular Medicine*. New York: Churchill Livingstone, 1995, pp. 1182–1187.

Furchgott, R. F., and Zawadzki, J. V. "The Obligatory Role of Endothelial Cells in the Relaxation of Arterial Smooth Muscle by Acetylcholine." *Nature*, 288 (1990) 373–376.

Galle, J.; Bassenge, E.; and Busse, R. "Oxidized Low Density Lipoproteins

Potentiate Vasoconstriction to Various Agonists by Direct Interaction with Vascular Smooth Muscle." *Circulation Research,* 66 (1990) 1287–1293.

Galle, J.; Mulsch, A.; Busse, R.; and Bassenge, E. "Effects of Native and Oxidized Low Density Lipoproteins on Formation and Inactivation of Endothelium-Derived Relaxing Factor." *Atheriosclerosis and Thrombosis,* 11 (1991) 198–203.

Gally, J. A.; Montague, P. R.; Reeke, G. N.; and Edelman, G. M. "The NO Hypothesis: Possible Effects of a Short-Lived, Rapidly Diffusible Signal in the Development and Function of the Nervous System." *Proceedings of the National Academy of Sciences, (USA),* 87 (1990) 3547–3551.

Garber, A. M.; Browner, W. S.; and Hulley, S. B. "Cholesterol Screening in Asymptomatic Adults, Revisited." *Annals of Internal Medicine,* 124 (1996) 518–531.

Garlick, P. J., and McNurlan, M. A. "Protein Metabolism in Cancer Patients." *Biochimie,* 76 (1994) 713–717.

Genis, P.; Jett, M.; Bernton, E. W.; Boyle, T.; Gelbard, A. A.; Dzenko, K.; Keane, R. W.; Resnick, L.; Mizrachi, Y.; Vosky, D. J.; Epstein, L. G.; and Gendelman, H. E. "Cytokines and Arachidonic Metabolites Produced during Human Immunodeficient Virus (HIV)-Infected Macrophage-Astroglia Interactions: Implications for the Neuropathogenesis of HIV Disease." *The Journal of Experimental Medicine,* 176 (1992) 1703–1718.

Gerlach, H.; Pappert, D.; Lewandowski, K.; Rossaint, R.; and Falke, K. J. "Long-Term Inhalation with Evaluated Low Doses of Nitric Oxide for Selective Improvement of Oxygenation in Patients with Adult Respiratory Distress Syndrome." *Intensive Care Medicine,* 19 (1993) 443–449.

Giannini, A. J.; Castellani, S.; and Dvoredsky, A. E. "Anxiety States: Relationship to Athmospheric Cations and Serotonin." *Journal of Clinical Psychiatry,* 44 (1983) 262–264.

Giannini, A. J.; Malone, D. A.; and Piotrowski, T. A. "The Serotonin Irritation Syndrome—A New Clinical Entity?" *Journal of Clinical Psychiatry,* 47 (1986) 22–25.

Gibbs, C. J.; Joy, A.; Heffner, R.; Franko, M.; Miyazaki, M.; Asher, D. M.; Parisi, J. E.; Brown, P. W.; and Gajdusek, D. C. "Clinical and Pathological Features and Laboratory Confirmation of Creutzfeldt-Jakob Disease in a Recipient of Pituitary-Derived Growth Hormone." *The New England Journal of Medicine,* 313 (1985) 734–738.

Giovannoni, G.; Heales, S. J. R.; Silver, N. C.; O'Riordan, J.; Miller, R. F.; Land, J. M.; Clark, J. B.; and Thompson, E. J. "Raised Serum Nitrate and Nitrite Levels in Patients with Multiple Sclerosis." *Journal of Neurological Sciences,* 145 (1997) 77–81.

Goldman, A. P.; Rees, P. G.; and Macrae, D. J. "Is It Time to Consider Domicilary Nitric Oxide?" *The Lancet,* 345 (1995) 199–200.

Gomaa, A.; Shalaby, M.; Osman, M.; Eissa, M.; Eizat, A.; Mahmoud, M.; and Mikhail, N. "Topical Treatment of Erectile Dysfunction: Randomized Double-Blind Placebo-Controlled Trial of Cream Containing Aminophylline, Isosorbide, and Co-Dergonic Mesulate." *British Medical Journal,* 312 (1996) 1512–1515.

Gordon, L. "L-Arginine May Help Reverse Age-Related Blood Vessel Damage." *The Medical Tribune,* 36 (1995) 4.

Gordon, T., and Kannel, W. B. "The Framingham, Massachusetts, Study Twenty Years Later." In Kessler, I. I., and Levin, M. L., eds., *The Community as an Epidemiologic Laboratory: A Casebook of Community Studies.* Baltimore: The Johns Hopkins University Press, 1970.

Gorfine, S. R. "Topical Nitroglycerin Therapy for Anal Fissures and Ulcers." *The New England Journal of Medicine,* 333 (1995) 1156–1157.

———. "Treatment of Benign Anal Disease with Topical Nitroglycerin." *Diseases of the Colon & Rectum,* 38 (1995) 453–457.

Green, L. C.; Ruiz De Luzuriaga, K.; Wagner, D. A.; Rand, W.; Istfan, N.; Young, V. R.; and Tannenbaum, S. R. "Nitrate Biosynthesis in Man." *Proceedings of the National Academy of Sciences (USA),* 78 (1981) 7764–7768.

Green, S. J., and Nacy, C. A. "Antimicrobial and Immunopathologic Effects of Cytokine-Induced Nitric Oxide Synthesis." *Current Opinion in Infectious Diseases,* 6 (1993) 384–396.

Grundy, S., chair, Task Force on Risk Reduction, "Cholesterol Screening in Asymptomatic Adults." *Circulation,* 93 (1996) 1067–1068.

Hamid, Q.; Springall, D. R.; Riveros-Moreno, V.; Chanez, P.; Horwath, P.; Redington, A.; Bousquet, J.; Godard, P.; Holgate, S.; and Polak, J. M. "Induction of Nitric Oxide Synthase in Asthma." *The Lancet,* 342 (1993) 1510–1513.

Hammond, G. L. "Endogenous Steroid Levels in the Human Prostate from Birth to Old Age: Comparison of Normal and Diseased Tissue." *Journal of Endocrinology,* 78 (1978) 7–15.

Hammond, I. W.; Devereux, R. B.; Alderman, M. H., et al. "The Prevalence and Correlates of Echocardiographic Left Ventricular Hypertrophy among Employed Patients with Uncomplicated Hypertension." *Journal of the American College of Cardiology,* 7 (1986) 639–650.

Hamon, M.; Valet, B.; Bauters, C.; Wenert, N.; McFadden, E. P.; Lablanche, J.-M.; Dupuis, B.; and Bertrand, M. "Long-Term Oral Administration of

L-Arginine Reduces Intimal Thickening and Enhances Neoendothelium-Dependent Acetylcholine-Induced Relaxation after Arterial Injury." *Circulation,* 90 (1994) 1357–1362.

Hanington, E. "The Platelet Theory." In Blau, J. N., ed. *Migraine.* Baltimore: The Johns Hopkins University Press, 1987, 265–302.

Hankey, B. "Breast Cancer in Younger Women: Strategies for Future Research." Bethesda, Md.: National Cancer Institute. Cited in Laurence, L., and Weinhouse, B. *Outrageous Practices.* New York: Fawcett Columbine, 1994, p. 117.

Harrison, D. G.; Armstrong, M. L.; Freiman, P. C.; and Heistad, D. D. "Restoration of Endothelium-Dependent Relaxation by Dietary Treatment of Atherosclerosis." *Journal of Clinical Investigation,* 80 (1987) 1808–1811.

Harvard Health Letter, vol. 18, 1993: Much Ado about NO, p. 6–7.

Heaton, J. P. W.; Morales, A.; Owen, J.; Saunders, F. W.; and Fenemore, J. "Topical Glyceryltrinitrate Causes Measurable Penile Arterial Dilation in Impotent Men." *The Journal of Urology,* 143 (1990) 729–731.

Hebert, P. R.; Fiebach, N. H.; Ebwerlein, K. A.; Taylor, J. O.; and Hennekens, C. H. "The Community-Based Randomized Trials of Pharmacologic Treatment of Mild-to-Moderate Hypertension." *American Journal of Epidemiology,* 127 (1988) 581–590.

Heitzer, T.; Just, H.; and Munzel, T. "Antioxidant Vitamin C Improves Endothelial Dysfunction in Chronic Smokers." *Circulation,* 94 (1996) 6–9.

Helmbrecht, G. D.; Farhat, M. Y.; Lochbaum, L.; Brown, H. E.; Yadgarova, K. T.; Eglinton, G. S.; and Ramwell, P. W. "L-Arginine Reverses the Adverse Pregnancy Changes Induced by Nitric Oxide." *American Journal of Obstetrics and Gynecology,* 175 (1996) 800–805.

Herbert, V. "Laetrile: The Cult of Cyanide Promoting Poison for Profit." *The American Journal of Clinical Nutrition,* 32 (1979) 1121–1158.

Hertz, P., and Richardson, J. A. "Arginine Induced Hyperkalemia." *Archives of Internal Medicine,* 130 (1972) 778–780.

Hibbs, J. B.; Vavrin, Z.; and Taintor, R. R. "L-Arginine Is Required for Expression of the Activated Macrophage Effector Mechanism Causing Selective Metabolic Inhibition in Target Cells." *The Journal of Immunology,* 138 (1987) 550–565.

Hirooka, Y.; Egashira, K.; Imaizumi, T.; Tagawa, T.; Kai, H.; Sugimashi, M.; and Takeshita, A. "Effects of L-Arginine on Acetylcholine-Induced Endothelium-Dependent Vasodilation Differs between the Coronary and Forearm Vasculatures in Humans." *Journal of the American College of Cardiology,* 24 (1994) 948–955.

Hishikawa, K.; Nakaki, T.; Suzuki, H.; Kato, R.; and Saruta, T. "L-Arginine as an Antihypertensive Agent." *Journal of Cardiovascular Pharmacology*, Supplement 12 (1992) 20, S196–S197.

Hishikawa, K.; Nakaki, T.; Tsuda, M.; Esumi, H.; Ohshima, H.; Suzuki, H.; Saruta, T.; and Kato, R. "Effect of Systemic L-Arginine Administration on Hemodynamics and Nitric Oxide Release in Man." *Japan Heart Journal*, 33 (1992) 41–48.

Hoffman, M. "A New Role for Gases: Neurotransmission." *Science*, 252 (1991) 1788.

Hofkelt, T.; Johansson, O.; Ljungdahl, A.; Lundberg, J. M.; and Schultzberg, M. "Peptidergic Neurons." *Nature*, 284 (1980) 515–521.

Hogaboam, C. M.; Jacobson, K.; Collins, S. M.; and Blennerhassett, M. G. "The Selective Beneficial Effects of Nitric Oxide Inhibition in Experimental Colitis." *American Journal of Physiology*, 268 (1995) G673–G684.

Hogan, J. C.; Lewis, M. J.; and Henderson, A. H. "In Vivo EDRF Activity Influences Platelets Function." *British Journal of Pharmacology*, 94 (1988) 1020–1022.

Hogg, N.; Struck, A.; Goss, S. P. A.; Santanam, N.; Joseph, J.; Parthasarathy, S.; and Kalyanaraman, B. "Inhibition of Macrophage-Dependent Low Density." *Journal of Lipid Research*, 36 (1993) 1756–1762.

Holden, C. "Lasker Awards." *Science*, 274 (1996) 39.

Hurson, M.; Regan, M. C.; Kirk, S. J.; Wasserkrug, H. L.; and Barbul, A. "Metabolic Effects of Arginine in a Healthy Elderly Population." *Journal of Parenteral & Enteral Nutrition*, 19 (1995) 227–230.

Iadecola, C. "Regulation of the Cerebral Microcirculation during Neural Activity: Is Nitric Oxide the Missing Link?" *Trends in Neurosciences*, 16 (1993) 206–214.

Iadecola, C.; Zhang, F.; and Xu, X. "Inhibition of Inducible Nitric Oxide Synthase Ameliorates Cerebral Ischemic Damage." *American Journal of Physiology*, 268 (1995) R286–R292.

Ialenti, A.; Ianaro, A.; Moncada, S.; and Di Rosa, M. "Modulation of Acute Inflammation by Endogenous Nitric Oxide." *European Journal of Pharmacology*, 211 (1992) 177–182.

Ialenti, A.; Moncada, S.; and Di Rosa, M. "Modulation of Adjuvant Arthritis by Endogenous Nitric Oxide." *British Journal of Pharmacology*, 110 (1993) 701–706.

Isidori, A.; Lo Monaco, A.; and Cappa, M. "A Study of Growth Hormone Release in Man after Oral Administration of Amino Acids." *Current Medical Research and Opinion*, 7 (1981) 475–481.

Izumi, H.; Yallampalli, C.; and Garfield, R. E. "Gestational Changes in L-Arginine-Induced Relaxation of Pregnant Rat and Human Myometrial Smooth Muscle." *American Journal of Obstetrics and Gynecology,* 169 (1993) 1327–1337.

Janovic, U. J., in Wagner, G., and Green, R. *Impotence—Physiological, Psychological, Surgical Diagnosis and Treatment.* New York: Plenum Press, 1981.

Jeremy, R. W.; McCarron, H.; and Sullivan, D. "Effects of Dietary L-Arginine on Atherosclerosis and Endothelium-Dependent Vasodilation in the Hypercholesterolemic Rabbit: Response According to Treatment Duration, Anatomic Site, and Sex." *Circulation,* 94 (1996) 498–506.

Jeserich, M.; Munzel, T.; Just, H.; and Drexler, H. "Reduced Plasma L-Arginine in Hypercholesterolaemia." *The Lancet,* 339 (1992) 561.

Joffe, I. I.; Travers, K. E.; Perreault, C. L.; Hamptom, T. G.; Katz, S. E.; Morgan, J. P.; and Douglas, P. S. "Impaired Nitric Oxide Availability Contributes to the Cardiac Dysfunction of Diabetes." *Circulation* (abstracts), 96 (1997) I518.

Johnson, A. W.; Land, J. M.; Thompson, E. J.; Bolanos, J. P.; Clark, J. B.; and Heales, S. J. R. "Evidence for Increased Nitric Oxide Production in Multiple Sclerosis." *Journal of Neurology, Neurosurgery, and Psychiatry,* 58 (1995) 107–115.

Johnson, C. L.; Rifkind, B. M.; Sempos, C. T.; Carroll, M. D.; Bachorik, P. S.; Briefel, R. R.; Gordon, D. J.; Burt, V. L.; Brown, C. D.; Lippel, K.; and Cleeman, J. I. "Declining Serum Total Cholesterol Levels among U.S. Adults: The National Health and Nutrition Examination Survey." *Journal of the American Medical Association,* 269 (1993) 3002–3008.

Johnstone, M. T.; Creager, S. J.; Scales, K. M.; Cusco, J. A.; Lee, B. K.; and Creager, M. A. "Impaired Endothelium-Dependent Vasodilation in Patients with Insulin-Dependent Diabetes Mellitus." *Circulation,* 88 (1993) 2510–2516.

Joint National Committee. "The 1988 Report of the Joint National Committee on Detection, Evaluation, and Treatment of High Blood Pressure." *Archives of Internal Medicine,* 148 (1988) 1023–1038.

Jorgensen, J. O. L.; Pedersen, S. A.; Thuesen, L.; Jorgensen, J.; Ingemann-Hansen, T.; Skakkebaek, N. E.; and Christiansen, J. S. "Beneficial Effects of Growth Hormone Treatment in GH-Deficient Adults." *The Lancet,* 1 (1989) 1221–1224.

Jover, B.; Herizi, A.; Ventre, F.; Dupont, M.; and Mimran, A. "Sodium and Angiotensin in Hypertension Induced by Long-Term Nitric Oxide Blockade." *Hypertension,* 21 (1993) 944–948.

Kamata, K.; Miyata, N.; and Kasuya, Y. "Impairment of Endothelium-Dependent Relaxation and Changes in Levels of Cyclic GMP in Aorta from Streptozotocin-Induced Diabetic Rats." *British Journal of Pharmacology*, 97 (1989) 614–618.

Kannel, W. B.; Castelli, W. P.; and McNamara, P. M. "Detection of the Coronary-Prone Adult: The Framingham Study." *Journal of the Iowa Medical Society*, 56 (1966) 26–34.

Kannel, W. B.; Castelli, W. P.; McNamara, P. M.; McKee, P. A.; and Feinleib, M. "Role of Blood Pressure in the Development of Congestive Heart Failure: The Framingham Study." *The New England Journal of Medicine*, 287 (1972) 781–787.

Kannel, W. B.; Gordon, T.; and Offutt, D. "Left Ventricular Hypertrophy by Electrocardiogram: Prevalence, Incidence and Mortality in the Framingham Study." *Annals of Internal Medicine*, 71 (1969) 89–105.

Kaplan, R. M. "Behavior as the Central Outcome in Health Care." *The American Psychologist*, 45 (1990) 1211–1220.

Kaplan, R. M.; Sallis, J. F.; and Patterson, T. L. *Health and Human Behavior.* New York: McGraw Hill, 1993.

Katusic, Z. S. "Superoxide Anion and Endothelial Regulation of Arterial Tone." *Free Radical Biology & Medicine*, 20 (1996) 443–448.

Katz, I. R. "Is There a Hypoxic Affective Syndrome?" *Psychosomatics*, 23 (1982) 846–853.

Kaur, H., and Halliwell, B. "Evidence for Nitric Oxide-Mediated Oxidative Damage in Chronic Inflammation: Nitrotyrosine in Serum and Synovial Fluid from Rheumatoid Patients." *Federation of European Biochemical Societies*, 350 (1994) 9–12.

Keller, R.; Geiges, M.; and Keist, R. "L-Arginine-Dependent Reactive Nitrogen Intermediates as Mediators of Tumor Cell Killing by Activated Macrophages." *Cancer Research*, 50 (1990) 1421–1425.

Kelly, E.; Morris, S. M.; and Billard, T. R. "Nitric Oxide, Sepsis, and Arginine Metabolism." *Journal of Parenteral & Enteral Nutrition*, 19 (1995) 234–238.

Kelly, J. P.; Kaufman, D. W.; Jurgeon, J. M.; Sheehan, J.; Koff, R. S.; and Shapiro, S. "Risk of Aspirin-Associated Major Upper Gastrointestinal Bleeding with Enteric Coated or Buffered Product." *The Lancet*, 348 (1996) 1413–1416.

Khaidar, A.; Marx, M.; Lubec, B.; and Lubec, G. "L-Arginine Reduces Heart Collagen Accumulation in the Diabetic dh/db Mouse." *Circulation*, 90 (1994) 479–483.

Kharitonov, S. A.; Lubec, G.; Hjelm, M.; and Barnes, P. J. "L-Arginine Increases Exhaled Nitric Oxide in Normal Human Beings." *Clinical Sciences*, 88 (1995) 135–139.

Kharitonov, S. A.; O'Connor, B. J.; Evans, D. J.; and Barnes, P. J. "Allergen-Induced Late Asthmatic Reactions Are Associated with Exhaled Nitric Oxide." *American Journal of Respiratory and Critical Care Medicine*, 151 (1995) 1894–1899.

Kharitonov, S. A.; Robbins, R. A.; Yates, D.; Keatings, V.; and Barnes, P. "Acute and Chronic Effects of Cigarette Smoking on Exhaled Nitric Oxide." *American Journal of Respiratory and Critical Care Medicine*, 152 (1995) 602–612.

Kharitonov, S. A.; Yates, D.; Robbins, R. A.; Logan-Sinclair, R.; Shinebourne, E. A.; and Barnes, P. J. "Increased Nitric Oxide in Exhaled Air of Asthmatic Patients." *The Lancet*, 343 (1994) 133–135.

King, R. G.; Gude, N. M.; Di-Iulio, J. L.; and Brennecke, S. P. "Regulation of Human Placental Fetal Vessel Tone: Role of Nitric Oxide." *Reproduction, Fertility & Development*, 7 (1995) 1407–1411.

Kinsella, J. P., and Abman, S. H. "Efficacy of Inhalational Nitric Oxide Therapy in the Clinical Management of Persistent Pulmonary Hypertension of the Newborn." *Chest*, 105 (1994) 92S–94S.

Klag, M. J.; Ford, D. E.; Mead, L. A.; He, J.; Whelton, P. K.; Liang, K. Y.; and Levine, D. M. "Serum Cholesterol in Young Men and Subsequent Cardiovascular Disease." *The New England Journal of Medicine*, 328 (1993) 313–318.

Kluger, J. "Can We Stay Young?" *Time*, November 25, 1996, 88–98.

Knowles, R. G.; Palacios, M.; Palmer, R. M. J.; and Moncada, S. "Formation of Nitric Oxide from L-Arginine in the Central Nervous System: A Transduction Mechanism for Stimulation of the Soluble Guanylate Cyclase." *Proceedings of the National Academy of Sciences (USA)*, 86 (1989) 5159–5162.

Kochi, M.; Takeuchi, S.; Mizutani, T.; Mochizuki, K.; Matsumoto, Y.; and Saito, Y. "Antitumor Activity of Benzaldehyde." *Cancer Treatment Reports*, 64 (1980) 21–23.

Kolata, G. "Key Signal of Cells Found to Be a Common Gas." *The New York Times*, July 2, 1991, C1 and C6.

Korbut, R.; Bieron, K.; and Gryglewski, R. J. "Effect of L-Arginine on Plasminogen-Activator Inhibitor in Hypertensive Patients with Hypercholesterolemia." *The New England Journal of Medicine*, 328 (1993) 287–288.

Koshland, D. E. "The Molecule of the Year." *Science*, 258 (1992) 1861–1863.

Krahn, M. D.; Mahoney, J. E.; Eckman, M. H.; Trachtenberg, J.; Pauker, S. G.; and Detsky, A. S. "Screening for Prostate Cancer: A Decision Analytic View." *Journal of the American Medical Association*, 272 (1994) 773–780.

Krueger, A. P., and Smith, R. F. "The Biological Mechanisms of Air Ion Action II: Negative Air Ion Effects on the Concentration and Metabolism of 5-Hydroxytryptamine in the Mammalian Respiratory Tract." *The Journal of General Physiology*, 44 (1960) 269–276.

Kubota, A.; Meguid, M. M.; and Hitch, D. C. "Amino Acid Profiles Correlate Diagnostically with Organ Sites in Three Kinds of Malignant Tumors." *Cancer*, 69 (1992) 2343–2348.

Kuhn, D. M., and Arthur, R. E. "Interaction of Tryptophan Hydroxylase by Nitric Oxide: Enhancement by Tetrahydrobiopterin." *Journal of Neurochemistry*, 68 (1997) 1495–1502.

Kuiper, M. A.; Visser, J. J.; Bergmans, P. L. M.; Scheltens, P.; and Wolters, E. C. "Decreased Cerebrospinal Fluid Nitrate Levels in Parkinson's Disease, Alzheimer's Disease and Multiple System Atrophy Patients." *Journal of Neurological Sciences*, 121 (1994) 46–49.

Kuo, L.; Davis, M. J.; Cannon, M. S.; and Chilian, W. M. "Pathophysiological Consequences of Atherosclerosis Extended into the Coronary Microcirculation: Restoration of Endothelium-Dependent Response by L-Arginine." *Circulation Research*, 70 (1992) 465–476.

Kwon, N. S.; Stuehr, D. J.; and Nathan, C. F. "Inhibition of Tumor Cell Ribonucleotide Reductase by Macrophage-Derived Nitric Oxide." *Journal of Experimental Medicine*, 174 (1991) 761–767.

Landzberg, M. J.; Graydon-Baker, E. M.; Fernandes, S. M.; Goldhaber, S. Z.; Desantis, J. M.; Hill, N. S.; Atz, A. M.; Body, S. C.; and Wessel, D. L. "Continuous Domiciliary Inhaled Nitric Oxide for Severe Pulmonary Hypertension." *Circulation* (Supplement 1), 96 (1997) I-244.

Lange, P. H. "Is the Prostate Pill Finally Here?" *The New England Journal of Medicine*, 327 (1992) 1234–1236.

Larson, D. E. *Mayo Clinic Family Health Book*, 2nd edition. New York: William Morrow and Company, Inc., 1996.

Lassen, L. H.; Shina, M.; Christiansen, I.; Ulrich, V.; and Olesen, J. "Nitric Oxide Inhibition in Migraine." *The Lancet*, 349 (1997) 401–402.

Leary, W. E. "Finding Intrigues Sickle Cell Experts." *The New York Times*, April 23, 1996, p. C5.

Lees, C.; Campbell, S.; Jauniaux, E.; Brown, R.; Ramsay, B.; Gibb, D.; Moncada, S.; and Martin, J. F. "Arrest of Preterm Labour and Prolongation of Gestation with Glyceryl Trinitrate, a Nitric Oxide Donor." *The Lancet*, 343 (1994) 1325–1326.

Lepor, H.; Williford, W. O.; Barry, M. J.; Brawer, M. K.; Dixon, C. M.; Gormley, G.; Haakenson, C.; Machi, M.; Narayan, P.; and Padley, R. J. "The Efficacy of Terazosin, Finasteride, or Both in Benign Prostatic Hyperplasia." *The New England Journal of Medicine*, 335 (1996) 533–539.

Lerman, A.; McKinley, L.; Higano, S. T.; and Holmes, D. R. "Oral Chronic L-Arginine Administration Improves Coronary Endothelial Function in Humans." *Supplement to the Journal of the American College of Cardiology*, 29 (1997) 192A–193A.

Loevenhart, A. S.; Lorenz, W. F.; Martin, H. G.; and Malone, J. Y. "Stimulation of Respiration by Sodium Cyanid [*sic*] and Its Clinical Application." *Archives of Internal Medicine*, 92 (1918) 109–129.

Lubec, B.; Hayn, M.; Kitzmuller, E.; Vierhapper, H.; and Lubec, G. "L-Arginine Reduces Lipid Peroxidation in Patients with Diabetes Mellitus." *Free Radical Biology & Medicine*, 22 (1997) 355–357.

Luboinski, G.; Nagadowska, M.; and Pienkowski, T. "Preoperative Chemotherapy in Primarily Inoperable Cancer of the Breast." *European Journal of Surgery and Oncology*, 17 (1991) 603–607.

Ludmer, P. L.; Selwyn, A. P.; Shook, T. L.; Wayne, R. R.; Mudge, G. H.; Alexander, R. W.; and Ganz, P. "Paradoxical Vasoconstriction Induced by Acetylcholine in Atherosclerotic Coronary Arteries." *The New England Journal of Medicine*, 315 (1986) 1046–1051.

Lund, J. N., and Scholefield, J. H. "A Randomised, Prospective, Double-Blind Placebo-Controlled Trial of Glyceryl Trinitrate Ointment in Treatment of Anal Fissure." *The Lancet*, 349 (1997) 11–14.

Lund, J. N.; Armitage, N. C.; and Scholefield, J. H. "Use of Glyceryl Trinitrate Ointment in Treatment of Anal Fissure." *British Journal of Surgery*, 83 (1996) 776–777.

Lundberg, J. O. N.; Hellstrom, P. M.; Lundberg, J. M.; and Alving, K. "Greatly Increased Luminal Nitric Oxide in Ulcerative Colitis." *The Lancet*, 344 (1994) 1673–1674.

———. "Nitric Oxide in Ulcerative Colitis." *The Lancet*, 345 (1995) 449.

Lyall, F.; Young, A.; and Greer, I. A. "Nitric Oxide Concentrations Are Increased in the Fetoplacental Circulation in Preeclampsia." *American Journal of Obstetrics and Gynecology*, 173 (1995) 714–718.

Lyons, C. R. "Emerging Roles of Nitric Oxide in Inflammation." *Hospital Practice*, July 15, 1996, 69–86.

Marcus, A. J., and Broeckman, J. "Cell-Free Hemoglobin as an Oxygen Carrier Removes Nitric Oxide, Resulting in Defective Thromboregulation." *Circulation*, 93 (1996) 208–209.

Marcus, M. L.; Koyanagi, S.; Harrison, D. G.; Doty, D. B.; Hiratzka, L. F.; and Eastham, C. L. "Abnormalities in the Coronary Circulation that Occur as a Consequence of Cardiac Hypertrophy." *American Journal of Medicine*, 75, Supplement 3A (1983) 62–66.

Marletta, M. A.; Yoon, P. S.; Iyengar, R.; Leaf, C. D.; and Wishnok, J. S. "Macrophage Oxidation of L-Arginine to Nitrite and Nitrate: Nitric Oxide Is an Intermediate." *Biochemistry*, 27 (1988) 8706–8711.

Masters, W., and Johnson, V. *Human Sexual Inadequacy*. Little Brown & Co., 1970.

Masui'yama, K.; Ochiai, H.; Niwayama, S.; Tazawa, K.; and Fujimaki, M. "Inhibition of Experimental and Spontaneous Pulmonary Metastasis of Murine RCT(+)sarcoma by Cyclodextrin-Benzaldehyde." *Japanese Journal of Cancer Research (Gann)*, 78 (1987) 705–711.

Mattei, F. M.; Capnone, M.; and Acconcia, A. "Impiego dell'estratto di Serenoa Repens nel Trattamento Medico della Ipertrofia Prostatica Benigna." *Urologia*, 55 (1988) 547–552.

McCarthy, A. L.; Woolfson, R. G.; Raju, S. K.; and Poston, L. "Abnormal Endothelial Cell Function of Resistance Arteries from Women with Preeclampsia." *American Journal of Obstetrics and Gynecology*, 168 (1993) 1323–1330.

McCartney-Francis, N.; Allen, J. B.; Mizel, D. E.; Albina, J. E.; Xie, Q.; Nathan, C. F.; and Wahl, S. M. "Suppression of Arthritis by an Inhibitor of Nitric Oxide Synthase." *Journal of Experimental Medicine*, 178 (1993) 749–754.

McCully, K. S. *The Homocysteine Revolution*. New Canaan, Conn.: Keats Publishing Inc., 1997.

McKenna, M.; Wolfson, S.; and Kuller, L. "The Ratio of Ankle and Arm Arterial Pressure as an Independent Predictor of Mortality." *Atherosclerosis*, 87 (1991) 119–128.

Medical Research Council Working Party on Mild to Moderate Hypertension, W. S. Peart, chair. "Adverse Reactions to Bendrofluazide and Propranolol for the Treatment of Mild Hypertension." *The Lancet*, 2 (1981) 540–543.

Mehta, S.; Stewart, D. J.; Langleben, D.; and Levy, R. D. "Short-Term Pulmonary Vasodilation with L-Arginine in Pulmonary Hypertension." *Circulation*, 92 (1995) 1539–1545.

Meister, A. *Biochemistry of the Amino Acids*, 2nd edition, Vol. I. New York: Academic Press, 1965, pp. 204–207.

Meltzer, H. Y., and Lowy, M. T. "The Serotonin Hypothesis of Depression." In Meltzer, H. Y., ed., *Psychopharmacology: The Third Generation of Progress.* New York: Raven Press, 1987.

Merimee, T. J.; Burgess, J. A.; and Rabinowitz, D. "Arginine Infusion in Maturity-Onset Diabetes Mellitus." *The Lancet*, 1 (1996) 1300–1301.

Merimee, T. J.; Lillicrap, D. A.; and Rabinowitz, D. "Effect of Arginine on Serum Levels of Human Growth Hormone." *The Lancet*, 2 (1965) 668–670.

Merimee, T. J.; Rabinowitz, D.; Riggs, L.; Burgess, J. A.; Rimoin, D. L.; and McKusick, V. A. "Plasma Growth Hormone after Arginine Infusion." *The New England Journal of Medicine*, 267 (1967) 434–439.

Merrill, J. E.; Ignarro, L. J.; Sherman, M. P.; Melinek, J.; and Lane, T. E. "Microglial Cell Cytotoxicity of Oligodendrocytes Is Mediated through Nitric Oxide." *Journal of Immunology*, 151 (1993) 2132–2141.

Mersdorf, A.; Goldsmith, P. C.; Diederichs, W.; Padula, C. A.; Lue, T. F.; Fishman, I. J.; and Tanagho, E. A. "Ultrastructural Changes in Impotent Penile Tissue: A Comparison of 65 Patients." *The Journal of Urology*, 145 (1991) 749–758.

Meyhoff, H. H.; Rosenkilde, P.; and Bodker, A. "Non-Invasive Management of Impotence with Transcutaneous Nitroglycerin." *British Journal of Urology*, 69 (1992) 88–90.

Middleton, S. J.; Shorthouse, M.; and Hunter, O. J. "Increased Nitric Oxide Synthesis in Ulcerative Colitis." *The Lancet*, 341 (1993) 465–466.

Miller, D.; Waters, D. D.; Warnica, W.; Szlachcic, J.; Kreeft, J.; and Theroux, P. "Is Variant Angina the Coronary Manifestation of a Generalized Vasospastic Disorder?" *The New England Journal of Medicine*, 13 (1981) 763–766.

Mills, C. D. "Molecular Basis of 'Suppressor' Macrophages: Arginine Metabolism via the Nitric Oxide Synthase Pathway." *The Journal of Immunology*, 146 (1991) 2719–2723.

Milner, J. A., and Stepanovich, L. V. "Inhibitory Effect of Dietary Arginine on Growth of Ehrlich Ascite Tumor Cells in Mice." *Journal of Nutrition*, 109 (1979) 489–494.

Mishina, D.; Katsel, P.; Brown, S. T.; Gilberts, E. C. A., M.; and Greenstein, R. J. "On the Etiology of Crohn's Disease." *Proceedings of the National Academy of Sciences (USA)*, 93 (1996) 9816–9820.

Moertel, C. G.; Fleming, T. R.; Rubin, J.; Kvols, L. K.; Sarna, G.; Koch, R.; Currie, V. E.; Young, C. W.; Jones, S. E.; and Davignon, J. P. "A Clinical Trial of Amygdalin (Laetrile) in the Treatment of Human Cancer." *The New England Journal of Medicine*, 306 (1982) 201–206.

Moncada, S. "The L-Arginine/Nitric Oxide Pathway." *Acta Physiologica Scandinavica,* 145 (1992) 201–227.

Moncada, S., and Higgs, E. A., eds. *Nitric Oxide from L-Arginine: A Bioregulatory System.* Amsterdam: Elsevier Science Publishers, 1990.

Moncada, S.; Palmer, R. M. J.; and Higgs, E. A. "Nitric Oxide: Physiology, Pathophysiology, and Pharmacology." *Pharmacological Reviews,* 43 (1991) 109–142.

———. "The Discovery of Nitric Oxide as the Endogenous Nitrovasodilator." *Hypertension,* 12 (1988) 365–372.

Mugge, A.; Elwell, J. H.; Peterson, T. E.; Hofmeyer, T. G.; Heistad, D. D.; and Harrison, D. G. "Chronic Treatment with Polyethylene-Glycolate Superoxide Dismutase Partially Restores Endothelium-Dependent Vascular Relaxation in Cholesterol-Fed Rabbits." *Circulation Research,* 69 (1991) 1293–1300.

Multiple Risk Factor Intervention Trial Research Group. "Baseline Rest Electrocardiographic Abnormalities, Antihypertensive Treatment, and Mortality in the Multiple Risk Factor Intervention Trial." *American Journal of Cardiology,* 55 (1985) 1–15.

Myatt, L.; Brewer, A.; and Brockman, D. E. "The Action of Nitric Oxide in the Perfused Human Fetal-Placental Circulation." *American Journal of Obstetrics and Gynecology,* 164 (1991) 687–692.

Nagano, I.; Shapshak, P.; Yoshioka, M.; Xin, K.; Nakamura, S.; and Bradley, W. G. "Increased NADPH-Diaphorase Reactivity and Cytokine Expression in Dorsal Root Ganglia in Acquired Immunodeficiency Syndrome." *Journal of the Neurological Sciences,* 136 (1996) 117–128.

Nakaki, T.; Hishikawa, K.; Suzuki, H.; Saruta, T.; and Kato, R. "L-Arginine-Induced Hypotension." *The Lancet,* 336 (1990) 696.

Nava, E.; Palmer, M. J.; and Moncada, S. "Inhibition of Nitric Oxide Synthesis in Septic Shock: How Much Is Beneficial?" *The Lancet,* 338 (1991) 1555–1557.

Negelev, S. "Re: Topical Nitroglycerin: A Potential Treatment for Impotence." *The Journal of Urology,* 143 (1990) 586.

Newman, H. F., and Northrup, J. D. "Mechanism of Human Penile Erection: An Overview." *Urology,* 17 (1981) 399–408.

Newman, T. B., and Hulley, S. B. "Carcinogenicity of Lipid-Lowering Drugs." *Journal of the American Medical Association,* 275 (1996) 55–69.

"Nitric Oxide May Contribute to AIDS." *AIDS Weekly,* May 31, 1993, p. 18.

Nozaki, K.; Moskowitz, M. A.; Maynard, K. I.; Koketsu, N.; Dawson, T. M.; Bredt, D. S.; and Snyder, S. H. "Origin and Distribution of Immunoreactive Nitric Oxide Synthase-Containing Nerve Fibers in Cerebral Arteries." *Journal of Cerebral Blood Flow and Metabolism,* 13 (1993) 70–79.

O'Kelly, T.; Brading, A.; and Mortensen, N. "Nerve Mediated Relaxation of the Human Internal Anal Sphincter: The Role of Nitric Oxide." *Gut,* 34 (1993) 689–693.

Ochoa, J. B.; Udekwu, A. O.; Billiar, T. R.; Curran, R. D.; Cerra, F. B.; Simmons, R. L.; and Peitzman, A. B. "Nitrogen Oxide Levels in Patients after Trauma and during Sepsis." *Annals of Surgery,* 214 (1991) 621–626.

Ohara, Y.; Peterson, T. E.; and Harrison, D. G. "Hypercholesterolemia Increases Endothelial Superoxide Anion Production." *Journal of Clinical Investigation,* 91 (1993) 2546–2551.

Olesen, J.; Thomsen, L. L.; Lassen, L. H.; and Olesen, I. J. "The Nitric Oxide Hypothesis of Migraine and Other Vascular Headaches." *Cephalgia,* 15 (1994) 94–100.

Oliver, M. F. "Risks of Correcting the Risks of Coronary Disease and Stroke with Drugs." *The New England Journal of Medicine,* 306 (1982) 297–298.

Ornish, D. M. *Dr. Dean Ornish's Program for Reversing Heart Disease.* New York: Random House, 1990.

Owen, J. A.; Saunders, F.; Harris, C.; Fenemore, J.; Reid, K.; Surridge, D.; Condra, M.; and Morales, A. "Topical Nitroglycerin: A Potential Treatment for Impotence." *The Journal of Urology,* 141 (1989) 546–548.

Pagnotta, P.; Germano, G.; Filippo, G. G.; Rosano, G. M. C.; and Chierchia, S. L. "Oral L-Arginine Supplementation Improves Essential Arterial Hypertension." *Circulation* (Supplement I), 96 (1997) 3014.

Park, K. G. M.; Hayes, P. D.; Garlick, P. J.; Sewell, H.; and Eremin, O. "Stimulation of Lymphocyte Natural Cytotoxicity by L-Arginine." *The Lancet,* 337 (1991) 645–646.

Park, K. G. M.; Heys, S. D.; Blessing, K.; Kelly, P.; McNurlan, M. A.; Eremin, O.; and Garlick, P. J. "Stimulation of Human Breast Cancers by Dietary L-Arginine." *Clinical Science,* 82 (1992) 413–417.

Pearson, D., and Shaw, S. *Life Extension.* New York: Warner Books, Inc., 1983.

Pelton, R., and Overholser, L. *Alternatives in Cancer Therapy.* New York: Fireside/Simon & Schuster, 1994.

Pemberton, C. M.; Moxness, K. E.; German, M. J.; Nelson, J. K.; and Gastineau, C. F. *Mayo Clinic Diet Manual.* Toronto: B. C. Decker, 1981.

Pennington, J. A. T. *Food Values.* New York: Harper Perennial, 1989.

Pepke-Zaba, J.; Higenbottam, T. W.; Dinh-Xuan, A. T.; Stone, D.; and Wallwork, J. "Inhaled Nitric Oxide as a Cause of Selective Pulmonary Vasodilation in Pulmonary Hypertension." *The Lancet,* 338 (1991) 1173–1174.

Petros, A.; Bennett, D.; and Vallance, P. "Effects of Nitric Oxide Synthase Inhibitors on Hypotension in Patients with Septic Shock." *The Lancet*, 338 (1991) 1557–1558.

Pezza, V.; Bernardini, F.; Pezza, B.; and Curione, M. "Study of Supplemental Oral L-Arginine (SOA) in Hypertensive Treated with Enalapril (E) + Hydrochlorithiazide (H)." *American Journal of Hypertension (Abstracts)*, 10 (1997) 179A.

Pieper, G. M., and Peltier, A. "Amelioration by L-Arginine of a Dysfunctional Arginine/Nitric Oxide Pathway in Diabetic Endothelium." *Journal of Cardiovascular Pharmacology*, 25 (1995) 397–403.

Pieper, G. M.; Siebeneich, W.; and Dondlinger, L. A. "Short-Term Administration of L-Arginine Reverses Defective Endothelium-Dependent Relaxation and cGMP Generation in Diabetes." *European Journal of Pharmacology*, 317 (1996) 317–320.

Podjarny, E.; Ben-Chetrit, S.; Rathaus, M.; Korzets, Z.; Green, J.; Katz, B.; and Bernheim, J. "Pregnancy-Induced Hypertension in Rats with Adriamycin Nephropathy Is Associated with an Inadequate Production of Nitric Oxide." *Hypertension*, 29 (1997) 986–991.

Quyyumi, A. A.; Dakak, N.; Mulcahy, D.; Andrews, N. P.; Husain, S.; Panza, J. A.; and Cannon, R. O., III. "Nitric Oxide Activity in the Atherosclerotic Human Coronary Circulation." *Journal of the American College of Cardiology*, 29 (1997) 308–317.

Quyyumi, A. A.; Husain, S.; Mulcahy, D.; Andrews, N. P.; Mincemoyer, R.; Panza, J. A.; and Cannon, R. O. "Nitric Oxide Activity in the Human Coronary and Peripheral Circulation." *Circulation Supplement*, 92 (1995) I-796.

Radomski, M. W.; Palmer, R. M. J.; and Moncada, S. "An L-Arginine/Nitric Oxide Pathway Present in Human Platelets Regulates Aggregation." *Proceedings of the National Academy of Sciences (USA)*, 87 (1990) 5193–5197.

Rajfer, J.; Aronson, W. J.; Bush, P. A.; Dorey, F. J.; and Ignarro, L. J. "Nitric Oxide as a Mediator of Relaxation of the Corpus Cavernosum in Response to Nonadrenergic, Noncholinergic Neurotransmission." *The New England Journal of Medicine*, 326 (1992) 90–94.

Rector, T. S.; Bank, A. J.; Mullen, K. A.; Tchumperlin, L. K.; Sih, R.; Pillai, K.; and Kubo, S. H. "Randomized, Double-Blind, Placebo Controlled Study of Supplemental Oral L-Arginine in Patients with Heart Failure." *Circulation*, 93 (1996) 2135–2141.

Reece Smith, H.; Memon, A.; Smart, C. J.; and Dewbury, K. "The Value of Permixon in Benign Prostatic Hypertrophy." *British Journal of Urology*, 58 (1986) 36–40.

Remvikos, Y.; Beuzebok, A.; Zajedal, A.; Voillment, N.; Magdelenat, H.; and Pouillant, P. "Correlation of Pretreatment Proliferative Activity of Breast Cancer with Response to Cytotoxic Chemotherapy." *Journal of the National Cancer Institute,* 81 (1989) 1383–1387.

Reynolds, P. D.; Middleton, S. J.; Hansford, G. M.; and Hunter, J. O. "Nitric Oxide in Ulcerative Colitis." *The Lancet,* 345 (1995) 448.

Ridker, P. M.; Cushman, M.; Stampfer, M. J.; Tracy, R. P.; and Hennekens, C. H. "Inflammation, Aspirin, and the Risk of Cardiovascular Disease in Apparently Healthy Men." *The New England Journal of Medicine,* 336 (1997) 973–979.

Roberts, J. M., and Redman, C. W. G. "Pre-Eclampsia: More than Pregnancy-Induced Hypertension." *The Lancet,* 341 (1993) 1447–1451.

Rodgers, A.; Jack, W. J. L.; Hardman, P. D. J.; Kerr, G. R.; Chetty, U.; and Leonard, R. C. F. "Locally Advanced Breast Cancer: Report of Phase II Study and Subsequent Phase III Trials." *British Journal of Cancer,* 65 (1992) 761–765.

Rodgers, G. M.; Taylor, R. N.; and Roberts, J. M. "Preeclampsia Is Associated with a Serum Factor Cytotoxic to Human Endothelial Cells." *American Journal of Obstetrics and Gynecology,* 159 (1988) 908–914.

Rooke, T. W., and Hirsh, A. T. "Peripheral Vascular Disease." In Willerson, J. T., and Cohn, J. N., eds. *Cardiovascular Medicine.* New York: Churchill Livingstone, 1995, pp. 1162–1181; figure 7.62, p. 1169.

Rose, W. C. "The Amino Acid Requirements of Adult Man." *Nutritional Abstract Review,* 27 (1957) 631–647.

Rose, W. C.; Haines, W. J.; and Warner, D. T. "The Amino Acid Requirements of Man." *Journal of Biological Chemistry,* 206 (1954) 421–430; Table IV, p. 429.

Rosenberg, I. H.; Bengoa, J. M.; and Sitrin, M. D. "Nutritional Aspects of Inflammatory Bowel Disease." *Annual Review of Nutrition,* 5 (1985) 463–484.

Ross, R. "The Pathogenesis of Atherosclerosis—An Update." *The New England Journal of Medicine,* 314 (1986) 488–500.

———. "Cell Biology of Atherosclerosis." *Annual Review of Physiology,* 57 (1995) 791–804.

Rossaint, R.; Falke, K. J.; Lopez, F.; Slama, K.; Pison, U.; and Zapol, W. M. "Inhaled Nitric Oxide for the Adult Respiratory Distress Syndrome." *The New England Journal of Medicine,* 328 (1993) 399–405.

Rudman, D.; Feller, A. G.; Nagraj, H. S.; Gergans, G. A.; Lalitha, P. Y.; Goldberg, A.; Schlenker, R. A.; Cohn, L.; Rudman, I. W.; and Mattson,

D. E. "Effects of Human Growth Hormone in Men over 60 Years Old." *The New England Journal of Medicine,* 323 (1990) 1–6.

Ryan, S. M.; Waack, B. J.; Weno, B. L.; and Heistad, D. D. "Increases in Pulse Pressure Impair Acetylcholine-Induced Vascular Relaxation." *American Journal of Physiology (Heart & Circulation Physiology),* 37 (1995) H359–H363.

Sakurai, H.; Kohsaka, H.; Liu, M.-F.; Higashiyama, H.; Hirata, Y.; Kanno, K.; Saito, I.; and Miyasaka, N. "Nitric Oxide Production and Inducible Nitric Oxide Synthase Expression in Inflammatory Arthritides." *The Journal of Clinical Investigation,* 96 (1995) 2357–2363.

Salazar, F. J.; Alberola, A.; Pinilla, J. M.; Romero, J. C.; and Quesada, T. "Salt-Induced Increase in Arterial Pressure during Nitric Oxide Synthesis Inhibition." *Hypertension,* 22 (1993) 49–55.

Satsangi, J.; Rees, D.; and Jewell, D. "Nitric Oxide in Ulcerative Colitis." *The Lancet,* 345 (1995) 449.

Schmidt, H. H. H. W.; Warner, T. D.; Ishii, K.; Sheng, H.; and Murad, F. "Insulin Secretion from Pancreatic B Cells Caused by L-Arginine-Derived Nitrogen Oxides." *Science,* 255 (1992) 721–723.

Schouten, W. R.; Briel, J. W.; Auwerda, J. J. A.; and De Graaf, E. J. R. "Ischaemic Nature of Anal Fissure." *British Journal of Surgery,* 83 (1996) 63–65.

Schuman, E. M., and Madison, D. V. "A Requirement for the Intercellular Messenger Nitric Oxide in Long-Term Potentiation." *Science,* 254 (1991) 1503–1506.

Shabsigh, R.; Fishman, I. J.; and Scott, F. B. "Evaluation of Erectile Impotence." *Urology,* 32 (1988) 83–90.

Sheperd, J. T.; Luscher, T. F.; and G. Mancia. "Circulatory Regulation: Basic Considerations." In Willerson, J. T., and Cohn, J. N., eds. *Cardiovascular Medicine.* New York: Churchill Livingstone, 1995, 1053–1067.

Shuster, S.; Black, M. M.; and McVitie, E. "The Influence of Age and Sex on Skin Thickness, Skin Collagen and Density." *British Journal of Dermatology,* 93 (1975) 639–643.

Sies, H. "Strategies of Antioxidant Defense." *European Journal of Biochemistry,* 215 (1993) 213–219.

Siragusa, M.; Batolo, D.; and Schepis, C. "Anetoderma Secondary to the Application of Leeches." *International Journal of Dermatology,* 35 (1996) 226–227.

Sitbon, O.; Denjean, F.; Bwergeron, A.; Parent, F.; Azarian, R.; Herve, P.; Raffestin, B.; and Simnneau, G. "Inhaled Nitric Oxide as a Screening Vasodilator Agent in Primary Pulmonary Hypertension: A Dose-

Response Study and Comparison with Prostacyclin." *American Journal of Respiratory and Critical Care Medicine,* 151 (1996) 384–389.

Slag, M. F.; Morley, J. E.; Elson, M. K.; Trence, D. L.; Nelson, C. J.; Nelson, A. E.; Kinlaw, W. B.; Beyer, H. S.; Nuttall, F. Q.; and Shafer, R. B. "Impotence in Medical Clinic Outpatients." *Journal of the American Medical Association,* 249 (1983) 1736–1740.

Smoyer, W. E.; Brouhard, B. H.; Rassin, D. K.; and LaGrone, L. "Enhanced GFR Response to Oral Versus Arginine Administration in Normal Adults." *Journal of Laboratory and Clinical Medicine,* 118 (1991) 166–175.

Snyder, S. H., and Bredt, D. S. "Biological Roles of Nitric Oxide." *Scientific American,* May 1992, pp. 68–77.

Sodeman, W. A., and Sodeman, T. M. *Pathological Physiology* (sixth edition). Philadelphia: W. B. Saunders, 1979.

Sooranna, S. R.; Morris, N. H.; and Steer, P. J. "Placental Nitric Oxide Metabolism." *Reproduction, Fertility & Development,* 7 (1995) 1523–1531.

Spark, R. F.; White, A.; and Connolly, P. B. "Impotence Is Not Always Psychogenic." *Journal of the American Medical Association,* 243 (1980) 750–755.

Stamler, J. S. "Alzheimer's Disease—A Radical Vascular Connection." *Nature,* 380 (1996) 108–111.

Stamler, J. S.; Jia, L.; Eu, J. P.; McMahon, T. J.; Demchenko, I. T.; Bonaventura, J.; Gerbert, K.; and Piantadosi, C. A. "Blood Flow Regulation by S-Nitrosohemoglobin in the Physiological Oxygen Gradient." *Science,* 276 (1997) 2034–2036.

Stamler, J.; Wentworth, D.; and Neaton, J. "Is the Relationship between Serum Cholesterol and Risk of Premature Death from Coronary Heart Disease Continuous and Graded?" *Journal of the American Medical Association,* 256 (1986) 2823–2828.

Stock, R. W. "How One Man Confronted and Conquered Impotence." *The New York Times,* Thursday, February 6, 1997, C4.

Stolley, P. D.; Tonascia, J. A.; Tockman, M. S.; Sartwell, P. E.; Rutledge, A. H.; and Jacobs, M. P. "Thrombosis with Low-Estrogen Oral Contraceptives." *American Journal of Epidemiology,* 102 (1975) 197–208.

Stroes, E. S. G.; Koomans, H. A.; de Bruin, T. W. A.; and Rabelink, T. J. "Vascular Function in the Forearm of Hypercholesterolaemic Patients off and on Lipid-Lowering Medication." *The Lancet,* 346 (1995) 467–471.

Stuehr, D. J., and Marletta, M. A. "Mammalian Nitrate Biosynthesis: Mouse Macrophages Produce Nitrite and Nitrate in Response to *Escherichia coli* Lipopolysaccharide." *Proceedings of the National Academy of Sciences (USA),* 82 (1985) 7738–7742.

Surtees, R., and Heales, S. "A Rostrocaudal Gradient of Nitrate plus Nitrite Concentration in CSF." *Journal of Neurology, Neurosurgery & Psychiatry,* 62 (1997) 1001–1010.

Takeda, Y.; Tominaga, T.; Tei, N.; Kitamura, M.; Taga, S.; Murase, J.; Taguchi, T.; and Kiwatani, T. "Inhibitory Effect of L-Arginine on Growth of Rat Mammary Tumors Induced by 7,12-Dymethylbenz(a)anthracene." *Cancer Research,* 35 (1975) 2390–2393.

Talley, J. D., and Crawley, I. S. "Transdermal Nitrate, Penile Erection, and Spousal Headache." *Annals of Internal Medicine,* 103 (1985) 804.

Tanner J. M. "Human Growth Hormone." *Nature,* 237 (1972) 433–439.

Thomas, T.; Thomas, G.; McLendon, C.; Sutton, T.; and Mullan, M. "B-Amyloid-Mediated Vasoactivity and Vascular Endothelial Damage." *Nature,* 380 (1996) 168–171.

Tomohiro, A.; Kimura, S.; He, H.; Fujisawa, Y.; Nishiyama, A.; Kiyomoto, K.; Aki, Y.; Tamaki, T.; and Abe, Y. "Regional Blood Flow in Dahl-Iwai Salt-Sensitive Rats and the Effects of L-Arginine Supplementation." *American Journal of Physiology,* 272 (1997) R1013–R1019.

Tortora, G. J., and Anagnostakos, N. P. *Principles of Anatomy and Physiology* (fourth edition). New York: Harper & Row, Publishers, 1984.

Tsai, G. E., and Gastfriend, D. R. "Nitric Oxide-Induced Motor Neuron Disease in a Patient with Alcoholism." *The New England Journal of Medicine,* 332 (1995) 1036.

Tsao, P. S.; McEvoy, L. M.; Drexler, H.; Butcher, E. C.; and Cooke, J. P. "Enhanced Endothelial Adhesiveness in Hypercholesterolemia Is Attenuated by L-Arginine." *Circulation,* 89 (1994) 2176–2182.

Tuomainen, T.-P.; Salonen, R.; Nyyssonen, K.; and Salonen, J. "Cohort Study of Relation between Donating Blood and Risk of Myocardial Infarction in 2,682 Men in Eastern Finland." *British Medical Journal,* 314 (1997) 793–794.

Tyler, V. E. *Herbs of Choice.* New York: Pharmaceuticals Products Press, 1994.

Ulm, M. R.; Plockinger, B.; Pirich, C.; Gryglewski, R. J.; and Sinzinger, H. F. "Umbilical Arteries of Babies Born to Cigarette Smokers Generate Less Prostacyclin and Contain Less Arginine and Citrulline Compared with Those of Babies Born to Control Subjects." *American Journal of Obstetrics and Gynecology,* 172 (1995) 1485–1487.

U.S. Department of Health and Human Services, National Cholesterol Education Program of the National Heart, Lung, and Blood Institute. *So You Have High Blood Cholesterol . . .* Washington, D.C.: NIH Publication No. 89-2922, 1989.

Vallance, P.; Patton, S.; Bhagat, K.; MacAllister, R.; Radomski, M.; Moncada, S.; and Malinski, T. "Direct Measurement of Nitric Oxide in Human Beings." *The Lancet,* 346 (1995) 153–154.

Van de Voorde, J.; Vanderstichele, H.; and Leusen, I. "Release of Endothelium-Derived Relaxing Factor from Human Umbilical Vessels." *Circulation Research,* 60 (1987) 517–522.

Vincent, S. R. "Nitric Oxide and Arginine-Evoked Insulin Secretion." *Science,* 258 (1992) 1376–1378.

Virag, R.; Bouilly, P.; and Frydman, D. "Is Impotence an Arterial Disorder?" *The Lancet,* 1 (1985) 181–184.

Visek, W. J. "Arginine Needs, Physiological State and Usual Diets: A Reevaluation." *Journal of Nutrition,* 116 (1986) 36–46.

Wade, N. "No Nobel Prize This Year? Try Footnote Counting." *The New York Times,* October 7, 1997, p. F4.

Wagner, G., and Green, R. *Impotence—Physiological, Psychological, Surgical Diagnosis and Treatment.* New York: Plenum Press, 1981.

Wallace, A. M., and Grant, J. K. "Effect of Zinc on Androgen Metabolism in the Human Hyperplastic Prostate." *Biochemical Society Transactions,* 3 (1975) 540–542.

Ward, W. K.; Bolgiano, D. C.; McKnight, B.; Halter, J. B.; and Porte, D. "Diminished B Cell Secretory Capacity in Patients with Noninsulin-Dependent Diabetes Mellitus." *Journal of Clinical Investigation,* 74 (1984) 1318–1328.

Watson, S. J.; Kamm, M. A.; Nicholls, R. J.; and Phillips, R. K. S. "Topical Glyceryl Trinitrate in the Treatment of Chronic Anal Fissure." *British Journal of Surgery,* 83 (1996) 771–775.

Weil, A. *Natural Health, Natural Medicine.* New York: Houghton Mifflin, 1990.

Weiner, C.; Knowles, R. G.; and Moncada, S. "Induction of Nitric Oxide Synthase Early in Pregnancy." *American Journal of Obstetrics and Gynecology,* 171 (1994) 838–843.

Wennmalam, A.; Benthin, G.; Edlund, A.; Jungersten, L.; Kieler-Jensen, N.; Lundin, S.; Nathorst, U.; Peterson, A.-S.; and Waagstein, F. "Metabolism and Excretion of Nitric Oxide in Humans." *Circulation Research,* 73 (1993) 1121–1127.

Werbach, M. R. *Nutritional Influences on Illness* (second edition). Tarzana, Ca.: Third Line Press, 1993.

Werbach, M. R., and Murray, M. T. *Botanical Influences on Illness.* Tarzana, Ca.: Third Line Press, 1994, pp. 76–77.

Werns, S. W.; Walton, J. A.; Hsia, H. H.; Nabel, E. G.; Sanz, M. L.; and Pitt,

A. "Evidence of Endothelial Dysfunction in Angiographically Normal Coronary Arteries of Patients with Coronary Artery Disease." *Circulation*, 79 (1989) 287–291.

Whitaker, J. *Dr. Whitaker's Guide to Natural Healing*. Rocklin, Ca.: Prima Publishing, 1995.

Williams, D. J.; Vallance, P. J. T.; Neild, G. H.; Spencer, J. A. D.; and Imms, F. J. "Nitric Oxide-Mediated Vasodilation in Human Pregnancy." *American Journal of Physiology*, 272 (1997) (*Heart & Circulation Physiology*, Vol. 41).

Wilson, J. D., and Gloyna, R. E. "The Intranuclear Metabolism of Testosterone in the Accessory Organs of Reproduction." *Recent Progress in Hormone Research*, 26 (1970) 309–336.

Winsor, T., and Beckett, J. C. "Biological Effects of Ionized Air in Man." *American Journal of Physical Medicine*, 37 (1958) 83–89.

Wolf, A.; Zalpour, C.; Theilmeier, G.; Wang, B-Y.; Ma, A.; Anderson, B.; Tsao, P. S.; and Cooke, J. P. "Dietary L-Arginine Supplementation Normalizes Platelet Aggregation in Hypercholesterolemic Humans." *Journal of the American College of Cardiology*, 29 (1997) 479–485.

Wong, J. L., and Whitaker, D. J. "Depressive Mood States and Their Cognitive and Personality Correlates in College Students: They Improve over Time." *Journal of Clinical Psychology*, 49 (1993) 615–621.

Xu, C.; Glagov, S.; Zatina, M. A.; and Zarins, C. K. "Hypertension Sustains Plaque Progression Despite Reduction of Hypercholesterolemia." *Hypertension*, 18 (1991) 123–129.

Yallampalli, C.; Izumi, H.; Byam-Smith, M.; and Garfield, R. "An L-Arginine-Nitric Oxide-Cyclic Guanosine Monophosphate System Exists in the Uterus and Inhibits Contractility during Pregnancy." *American Journal of Obstetrics and Gynecology*, 170 (1993) 175–185.

Yates, D. H.; Kharitonov, S. A.; Robbins, R. A.; Thomas, P. S.; and Barnes, P. J. "Effect of a Nitric Oxide Synthase Inhibitor and a Glucocorticosteroid on Exhaled Nitric Oxide." *American Journal of Respiratory and Critical Care Medicine*, 152 (1995) 892–896.

Zangerle, R.; Fuchs, D.; Reibnegger, G.; Werner-Felmayer, G.; Gallati, H.; Wachter, H.; and Werner, E. R. "Serum Nitrite Plus Nitrate in Infection with Human Immunodeficiency Virus Type-1." *Immunobiology*, 193 (1995) 59–70.

Zeiher, A. M.; Drexler, H.; Wollschlager, H.; and Just, H. "Endothelial Dysfunction of the Coronary Microvasculature Is Associated with Impaired Coronary Blood Flow Regulation in Patients with Early Atherosclerosis." *Circulation*, 84 (1991) 1984–1992.

Zeiher, A. M.; Schachinger, V.; and Minners, J. "Long-Term Cigarette Smoking Impairs Endothelium-Dependent Coronary Arterial Vasodilator Function." *Circulation,* 92 (1995) 1094–1100.

Zhang, F.; White, J. G.; and Iadecola, C. "Nitric Oxide Donors Increase Blood Flow and Reduce Brain Damage in Focal Ischemia: Evidence that Nitric Oxide Is Beneficial in the Early Stages of Cerebral Ischemia." *Journal of Cerebral Blood Flow and Metabolism,* 14 (1994) 217–226.

Zhang, J., and Snyder, S. H. "Nitric Oxide in the Nervous System." *Annual Review of Pharmacology and Toxicology,* 35 (1995) 213–233.

Zorgniotti, A. W., and Lizza, E. F. "Effect of Large Doses of Nitric Oxide Precursor, L-Arginine, on Erectile Dysfunction." *International Journal of Impotence Research,* 6 (1994) 33–36.

INDEX

233